AROMATHERAPY FOR
Menopause SUCCESS

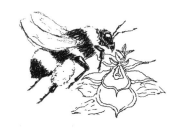

100 Essential Oil Recipes
to Reclaim Your Vibrancy

with love,

Angela

ANGELA SIDLO, CHA, CHC, CR

Aromatherapy for Menopause Success: 100 essential oil recipes to reclaim your vibrancy
Copyright 2018 Saddle Mt. Healing Arts Press

For information about special discounts for bulk purchases, speaking engagements or events contact Angela Sidlo at angela.sidlo@gmail.com or visit the www.AngelaSidlo.com

Printed in the United States of America

Library of Congress Control Number: 2018912453
ISBN: 978-1-7325625-0-9 (paperback)
ISBN 978-1-7325625-1-6 (e-book)

About the cover:
watercolor illustration and interior artwork by Patti Breidenbach
cover photo & author photo by Denise Faddis
original artist for logo inspiration Terrie Remington
logo graphic design by Morgan Wichman
cover & interior design by Amie Olson

Disclaimer:

The various uses of essential oils for health and wellness are based on traditional wisdom, scientific theories or limited research. Often times they have not been thoroughly tested for their safety and effectiveness in clinical trials. Some of the conditions where essential oils can be effective are potentially serious and should be discussed with a qualified medical practitioner. This book is intended educational purposes only, and should not be used to diagnose or treat any health condition. In light of the complex, bio-individual and specific nature of health problems, this book is not intended to replace professional medical advice. The ideas, procedures, and suggestions in this book are intended to compliment not replace the advice of a trained medical professional. Consult your physician before adopting any of the suggestions in this book as well as any conditions that may require diagnosis or medical attention. The author and publisher disclaim any liability arising directly or indirectly from the use of this book.

To all of the women around the world
who are looking to find balance
during this transitional time of your lives,
I dedicate this book to you.
May you discover peace, happiness and joy.

Contents

Acknowledgements

I'd like to thank the people who were instrumental in making my dream of this book become a reality. First and foremost, thank you to my husband Kirby who is the wind in my sails. Your support, love and kindness is beyond measure and I couldn't have achieved this much without you as my life partner. You are a blessing.

To Cristine Shade whose assistance, patience and computer wizardry I could not be without. You kept me calm when I felt like everything was falling apart.

Kudos to Amie Olson whose brilliant graphic design skills made this book so beautiful. You captured my ideas and made them come to life.

Thanks and hugs to Patti Breidenbach, your talent as an artist leaves me awe stricken. The clary sage watercolor for the cover is everything I had envisioned.

Thank you to my accountability partner, Katrina Touck'e and all of my friends who proofread, edited and challenged me to do better. To the hundreds of women who have tried my aromatherapy blends and found amazing results. Thank you for believing in me and encouraging me to move forward. Much gratitude to my little coastal community for supporting me as a holistic health practitioner by coming to my classes, talks and gatherings over the past 10 years to learn more and allow me to share.

I'd like to give utmost gratitude to all the medicinal plants for offering their life force energy as essential oils. These oils kept me uplifted, focused and energized as I researched, wrote and created recipes. They were constant companions showing me the way. My wish it that we can all continue to learn from the oils, together.

Introduction

For thousands of years throughout history women have used aromatic plants to usher their bodies into the wisdom years of menopause. This should be a beautiful time in your life where you finally have a chance to focus on yourself, honor your body and share your innate wisdom with others. It is actually the most exciting time of your life. Menopause is neither a diagnosis nor a disease! The symptoms of menopause are not normal and hormone replacement therapy can't offer sustainable solutions.

However, listening to your body, reducing your stress levels and making lifestyle changes with the use of essential oils can be powerful medicine. Our western culture views older women as less than the "wise women" that we truly are. It's time to rise up and change this perception. I believe essential oils can help in this effort by increasing your energy, showing your true inner beauty and giving you the radiance that all women deserve to experience.

My first experience with aromatic plant medicine began when my grandmother let me help in her rose garden. I was drawn to the sweet aromas of each rose as it blossomed. I felt safe, comforted and loved there. It wasn't until I was in my early 40's when I reconnected with those aromas in essential oils. I was in the early stages of peri-menopause. Plagued with anxiety, depression, bloating, heavy periods, brain fog and fatigue, I was desperate for answers. I began inhaling several essential oils on a regular basis and soon realized that my brain fog had diminished. I continued to improve and my anxiety and depression subsided. I started to feel more energy and knew that working with essential oils would become my path in life.

Aromatherapy is the fastest growing complementary healthcare modality in the 21st century. Yet misuse of essential oils due to a lack of proper education still exists. This book will give you safe, effective and proven information and formulas to help you balance hormones and experience renewed hope for easing through peri-menopause and menopause.

Over the past decade I have refined my knowledge and use of essential oils and focus solely on women's health and hormone balance as an aromatherapist, reflexologist and energy worker. Aromatherapy has transformed how I take care of my body on a daily basis. It bridges the gaps of my foundational lifestyle habits of nutrition, exercise, stress management, sleep and meditation.

Experiencing hormone imbalances has truly been a blessing for me. I know firsthand what my clients are experiencing and have created and tested the essential oil blends that bring the body back into balance.

With the use of essential oils you will be able to experience a paradigm shift and a new way of life. For many women, it is often the missing link to otherwise seemingly impossible challenges during their transition into menopause.

You are responsible for your own health care. Not a doctor, nurse practitioner, naturopath, insurance company or even another family member. With this book, I will teach you how to use essential oils to balance hormones and begin to take charge of your own health, naturally.

I believe we can look to nature for solutions to imbalances in the body. Nature is a good example of always achieving balance through the cycles of time to rejuvenate and renew. Essential oils can help you with the process of change and transformation through menopause.

In this book you'll understand how to use essential oils to help you holistically balance hormones on a body, mind and spirit level. You will be amazed at the changes you will experience through the information and recipes included here. I'll show you how hormones work in the body and the connection to the limbic system in the brain that enables essential oils to create chemical changes that affect us physically, mentally and emotionally. I'll share with you how to take control of your health and wellbeing. You will learn how to make simple yet powerful changes with the formulas I have created for you.

This book is my gift to you so that you may experience the benefits of balanced hormones including better memory, more energy, easing of hot flashes and night sweats, increased libido, less anxiety and depression and feeling more comfortable in your body.

I'm so very honored to share this first book with you in the Menopause Success series. Thank you for joining me on this journey into the world of essential oils for hormone balance.

Scentfully Yours,

Angela Sidlo

How To Use This Book

To get the most out of this book I have designed it to give you the science behind what's happening to your body along with specific guidance to use key essential oils that allow your body to find hormonal bliss. Yes, I'm a bit of a science geek so bear with me. I don't want this to be one of those books that sits on your shelf all nice and pretty. There are spaces for you to write notes, jot down your thoughts and record exactly what is happening to you in peri-menopause or menopause. I know that as a woman going through this stage of your life you can get irritated easily, experience brain fog and feel there is no hope. The last thing you want is a book that doesn't quickly give you answers to your problems.

Part 1 will explain what essential oils are, how they are produced and ways they interact with your endocrine system. Part 2 guides you through various hormones that get out of balance as you enter menopause. It will help you understand exactly what is going on. I created detailed checklists of symptoms and left you some space for notes. Part 3 introduces the Quick Reference Guides. These are real gems where you can quickly see which hormones are out of balance and the find the essential oils that offer solutions. Part 4 gives you 100 recipes that I have developed, adapted and used over the past 10 years in my own journey with peri-menopause and menopause. These recipes have been tested by myself and hundreds of the women I have worked with as an aromatherapist and health coach. To finish out the book there is an appendix that gives you the essential oil descriptions for a more in depth look at the hormone balancing properties of each essential oil used in this book.

Lastly I've included a resource list for you to find quality essential oils and ingredients to make your blends. As a true aromatherapist I believe in sourcing oils from small companies that take care in the purity of their product and providing it at a good pricing with no middle man. In my association with NAHA and my colleagues in the field of aromatherapy I have found some amazing purveyors of essential oils. I'm happy to share my sources with you so the you too can achieve optimal health just as I have.

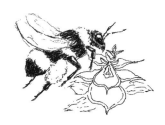

PART 1

Using Essential Oils for Hormone Balance

Having balanced hormones wasn't even on my radar when I was younger. I was in my late 30's running my own Italian restaurant and pasta manufacturing business. I started my 12 hour day with two shots of espresso, scrambled eggs and leftover pasta from the night before. I was working with wheat flour all day while manufacturing pasta for other local restaurants as well as my own. By mid afternoon I needed another pick me up as my energy levels and stamina waned. Two more shots of espresso and a slice of tiramisu and I was good to go. That's when the night sweats began and sleep became illusive. My joints ached and I was plagued with agitated depression, anxiety, panic attacks, headaches and bloating. My periods were painful and my sex drive hit an all time low. I truly thought I was going crazy. The last thing I considered was the possibility of my hormones being out of whack.

I decided it was time to see my allopathic doctor about what was going on. She sent me to a rheumatologist and a gynecologist. The rheumatologist diagnosed me with fibromyalgia and put me on a plethora of medications including anti-inflammatories, serotonin uptake inhibitors and antidepressants. The gynecologist wanted to put me on birth control to deal with the symptoms of painful periods and raging PMS. She also suggested that I use Crisco, yes Crisco as a vaginal lubricant! Needless to say I was seriously disappointed in the healthcare system and still suffering from symptoms that were making my daily life a living hell.

Not once did any of these doctors talk to me about my hormones or natural processes that happen to a woman throughout her reproductive years. Just to be clear, Menopause is the time of your life when you naturally stop having menstrual periods. It marks the end of our reproductive years. Since our periods can fluctuate during peri-menopause (the phase when the ovaries start to produce less estrogen), you know you've truly hit menopause after you go 12 months without a period.

I took the medications for a while but they left me feeling like a zombie and were only masking the underlying symptoms. Several years later with a lot of research and trial and error, I discovered more natural means of taking care of my body. I had actually been experiencing hormone imbalances related to chronic stress, peri-menopause and poor diet and lifestyle choices.

I discovered essential oils, meditation, reflexology and health coaching and a more holistic life emerged for me. I'm free from all of the previous symptoms that plagued me back then. I feel younger than ever, that's why I'm sharing this book with you as the first in the Menopause Success series so that you can learn natural ways to bring your body into the most beautiful, creative and fulfilling time of your life. Essential oils have played a major role in my recovery, relieving depression and anxiety, improving sleep, eliminating hot flashes and managing sugar cravings.

I don't want you to have to go through the frustration and pain that I did. I believe that finding true hormone balance in peri-menopause and menopause required a multifaceted approach that includes diet, lifestyle changes and supplements. As a health coach and aromatherapist, when I begin a conversation about balancing hormones with my clients, it all of this can seem very daunting and even unattainable. This is why I begin a comprehensive program with essential oils to help the body begin to balance on an emotional and physical level so that the tasks of making lifestyle and diet changes can be achieved. The effects of essential oils and their therapeutic benefits can boost confidence, reduce stress levels, support body systems and even aid in detoxification. Essential oils will always be my first "go to" for the body to begin to shift hormones back into balance.

I'll explain to you how your hormones work and who the major players are in peri-meno-pause and menopause. Hormones dominate every aspect of your daily life. They regulate literally hundreds of bodily functions. Mood, cravings, heart regulation, fluid balance and sex drive just to name a few. All of these functions are controlled by your hormones. If there isn't enough of one hormone or too much of another then things start to get a little wonky. That's where essential oils come to the rescue. They have the ability to communicate on a cellular level with your hormones to create the perfect remedy on the spot.

The use of essential oils for women's health encompasses virtually every culture on earth. The ancient Greeks used aromatic baths and massages to relieve women's health symptoms. Chinese medicine texts discuss the use of aromatics for women. Native Americans sought out the use of herbal and aromatic plants to nourish women through all of the phases of their lives. It is a part of our cultural heritage that we have forgotten. I hope to rekindle that which your body has forgotten and remind the precious feminine spirit within you of this ancient plant wisdom for healing.

Essential oils are natural aromatic compounds found in plants. They are found in the roots, seeds, stems, bark, leaves and flowers and are distilled and extracted for their therapeutic benefits. They are 50-70 times more concentrated than dried herbs. Essential oils contain dozens, if not hundreds of unique metabolites and organic chemical constituents. Our bodies do not develop resistances or intolerances to essential oils due to the organic chemical nature of essential oils. They work on a cellular level to create harmony in the body. Essential oils possess adaptogenic properties which means they help our bodies to adapt to changing conditions and manage stress. When our bodies experience an essential oil, it's like an orchestra full of musical instruments all playing the same piece of music. Everyone is in perfect harmony. Every essential oil in its purest form is also antiviral and antibacterial. With these properties they support our immune system which is an important part of hormone balance.

There are about 350 plants that provide essential oils that possess therapeutic qualities. The most common way to extract the oils is a process called distillation. Plant material is placed into a stainless steel or copper container. Water is introduced and heated to create a steam. The steam rises, extracting the oil. It then travels to a condenser where it is cooled. From there the oil separates from the liquid. The essential oil is the oily portion.

The liquid portion is called a hydrosol. Hydrosols are very useful in making spritzers and body care products and also have therapeutic value.

Citrus oils are harvested from the peel of the fruit through a cold press method. Other methods of extraction use solvents. I prefer oils produced through distillation and cold press for therapeutic benefits. To give you an example of how powerful an essential oil is, it takes 10,000 pounds of rose petals to produce 1 pound of rose essential oil using distillation. Each drop of rose oil is equivalent to 70 rose buds. That's powerful plant medicine! It also means that you only need to use 1 single drop to receive therapeutic benefits. So less is more.

How does all of this work in the body? Essential oils operate via the olfactory system which is your sense of smell. Every organ in your body possesses olfactory receptors. That doesn't mean every organ has the ability to smell but it does mean that every organ has the ability to interact and receive information from essential oils. When you smell an essential oil, it travels through the oldest part of the brain, the limbic system. There it is processed by the hypothalamus and sends out a cascade of chemistry that it interpreted on a mental, physical and emotional level by the body. For example; when you inhale lavender, the body sends out chemistry to the olfactory receptors in the spinal cord and endocrine system to calm your nervous system, relieve pain and balance hormones. All of this happens via olfactory receptors throughout the body.

Here is a chart that shows essential oil pathways in the body.

Olfactory Pathway into the Body

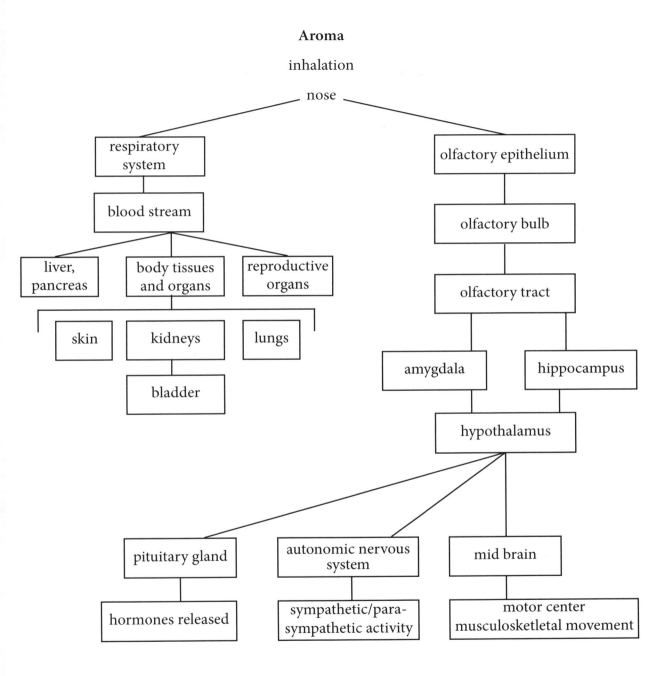

Aroma

inhalation

nose

respiratory system

blood stream

liver, pancreas

body tissues and organs

reproductive organs

skin

kidneys

lungs

bladder

olfactory epithelium

olfactory bulb

olfactory tract

amygdala

hippocampus

hypothalamus

pituitary gland

autonomic nervous system

mid brain

hormones released

sympathetic/para-sympathetic activity

motor center musculosketletal movement

Methods of application to use essential oils include inhalation, applying to the skin through massage, perfume, lotion, salve, body butter, foot soak, epsom salt bath or compress. As a holistic aromatherapist I do not recommend ingesting essential oils. The mucosal membranes in the mouth and digestive system are very fragile and essential oils can cause damage to this lining. I see people putting lemon essential oil in their water bottle to help alkalize. Oil and water don't mix! The oil goes straight onto your mucosal membranes without a carrier oil to bind it and it will damage the delicate tissues of your mouth, throat and esophagus. Even a drop of an essential oil such as peppermint on or under your tongue can cause damage. I do include recipes in this book for vaginal suppositories. These have a carrier oil with them so they will not burn your internal membranes and tissues. Always consult with a qualified practitioner if you are considering the use of essential oils internally.

Safety first! It is always my mission as a holistic aromatherapist, to provide individuals with information on the safe and effective use of essential oils. Here are some of my basic rules for safety.

- Keep all essential oils out of reach of children
- Avoid use of photosensitizing oils including citrus oils before exposure to sun
- Avoid use of undiluted essential oils on the skin
- Do a test patch on the skin prior to applying essential oils to a large area of skin
- If an oil causes a skin irritation, apply more carrier oil to the area
- Do not use essential oils internally (Always consult a professional)
- Use extreme caution when using essential oils during pregnancy (consult a professional first)
- Keep essential oils away from the eyes and other mucosal membranes
- Use essential oils in a well ventilated room
- Keep essential oils away from pets, especially cats and birds

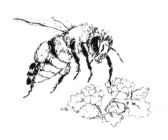

PART 2

Understanding Your Hormones

Hormones are produced by the endocrine system in the body. As with all body systems, it is very intricate. The endocrine system hormone producing and hormone synthesizing organs and glands includes the following:

- Pituitary Gland
- Pineal Gland
- Thyroid and Parathyroid Glands
- Heart
- Kidneys
- Adrenal Glands
- Stomach
- Pancreas
- Intestines
- Ovaries in Women
- Testes in Men

Each organ has a role to play but the system has to be coordinated in their efforts to keep the balance. There are a multitude of hormones produced by the endocrine system. I often wonder why western medical doctors don't look at hormone imbalances first when trying find relief for the symptoms of many illnesses. When hormones are out of balance it effects every other body system.

THE ENDOCRINE SYSTEM

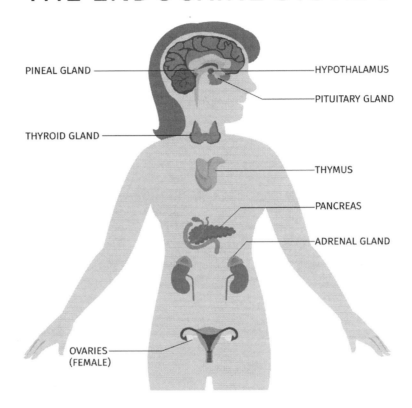

I'll focus on the top 5 Hormones major players regarding peri-menopause and menopause that effect most women.

1. **Estrogen**

2. **Progesterone**

3. **Cortisol**

4. **Insulin**

5. **Thyroid**

Some other hormones I consider to be minor league players, but equally important, are leptin, cholesterol and oxytocin but whether you are the pitcher or the left field player, it takes a team that works together in harmony to win the game. There are many other hormones at work in the endocrine system. Here is a chart that gives you a bigger picture.

HORMONES

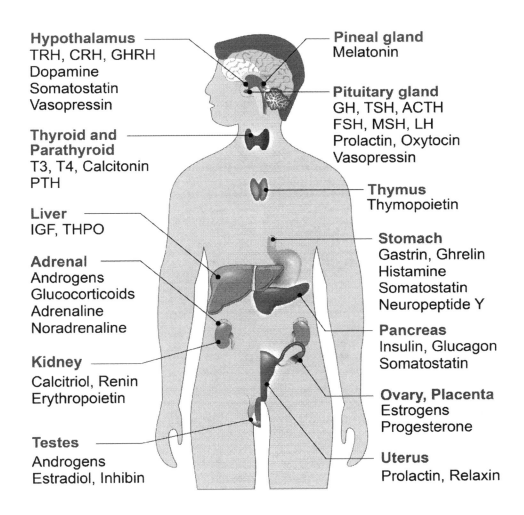

Hypothalamus
TRH, CRH, GHRH
Dopamine
Somatostatin
Vasopressin

Thyroid and Parathyroid
T3, T4, Calcitonin
PTH

Liver
IGF, THPO

Adrenal
Androgens
Glucocorticoids
Adrenaline
Noradrenaline

Kidney
Calcitriol, Renin
Erythropoietin

Testes
Androgens
Estradiol, Inhibin

Pineal gland
Melatonin

Pituitary gland
GH, TSH, ACTH
FSH, MSH, LH
Prolactin, Oxytocin
Vasopressin

Thymus
Thymopoietin

Stomach
Gastrin, Ghrelin
Histamine
Somatostatin
Neuropeptide Y

Pancreas
Insulin, Glucagon
Somatostatin

Ovary, Placenta
Estrogens
Progesterone

Uterus
Prolactin, Relaxin

I want to break down each one of the five major hormones so you can really get a better understanding of what is happening to your body. I often compare the feelings of menopause to reflections of puberty. We begin to notice subtle changes in our bodies that make us feel uncomfortable, self conscious and sometimes unworthy. Remember what it was like when you started developing breasts? You felt self conscious and awkward. Reflect on one of the aspects of how your body is changing now. What feelings come up? Are you feeling those same uncomfortable feelings you had as a young teen? These symptoms can catch us by surprise and change who we are and how we feel about ourselves and the shifts our bodies are experiencing. Not to mention how our current culture begins to view us as we age. I want to give you information that will help you realize first of all that you are not alone and secondly, that all of this is something that can be sorted out so you can get back to feeling good in your own skin again.

Let's take a look at what estrogen and progesterone are doing throughout the cycle of your life. I wish the nuns that my mother sent me to at the catholic church when I reached puberty had explained this. I remember they were teaching a class to young girls about puberty, starting your period and sex. I was eleven and my mother made sure I was there. As I sat in class listening to them explain how your uterus is about the size of a pear and forming my hand to look like a pear, I thought to myself, "What do nuns know about all of this, they're not even supposed to have sex!" I questioned a lot of things as a young girl. Sometimes that got me into trouble but I feel that it gave me the courage and tenacity to help you find the answers you deserve, especially when it comes to knowing what your body is going through.

During a woman's reproductive years, roughly from your teens to early forties, your estrogen and progesterone levels should stay evenly distributed. During peri-menopause estrogen levels are all over the board giving you a wild ride of mood swings and emotional upheaval. Progesterone begins to dramatically decline during this time as well. In menopause, both estrogen and progesterone ride off into the sunset leaving you to experience a myriad of symptoms physically, mentally and emotionally.

One third of a woman's life is spent in some stage of menopause! (peri-menopause, menopause, post-menopause) Wouldn't you love to spend this time of your life loving the body you live in, being inspired as a wise woman and standing in your own power?

Estrogen and Progesterone Levels Throughout a Woman's Life

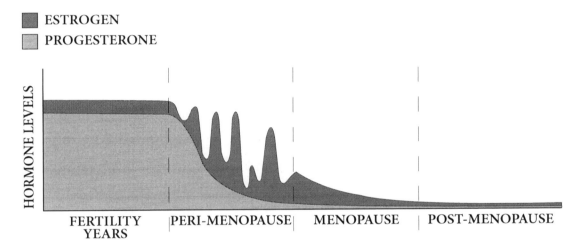

■ ESTROGEN
□ PROGESTERONE

HORMONE LEVELS

FERTILITY YEARS | PERI-MENOPAUSE | MENOPAUSE | POST-MENOPAUSE

Monthly Menstrual Cycle Estrogen/Progesterone Levels

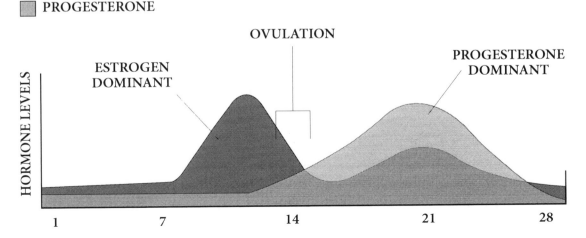

■ ESTROGEN
□ PROGESTERONE

HORMONE LEVELS

ESTROGEN DOMINANT

OVULATION

PROGESTERONE DOMINANT

1   7   14   21   28

During a woman's reproductive years her monthly menstrual cycle has its own unique estrogen/progesterone carnival roller coaster. I'm sure you have purchased tickets for this ride without even knowing it. The bonuses include free mood swings, wild sugar cravings, irritability, fatigue and so much more! Seriously, this can be a real challenge for many women even into menopause. Using essential oils can definitely negotiate these symptoms and help your body gracefully step off the roller coaster ride.

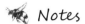 *Notes*

Understanding Estrogen

Estrogen can be one of the most misunderstood hormones that cause women the most grief during peri-menopause and menopause. I'll break it down and then share some essential oils that can help you keep the balance.

Estrogen is the hormone that dominates the female body. It isn't a single biological compound though. In fact, there are several forms of this hormone. The three primary forms are estrone (E1) weaker estrogen that is higher in menopausal women, estradiol (E2) often referred to as antagonistic estrogen and estriol (E3) protective estrogen. If that isn't confusing enough, there are also phytoestrogens (estrogen-like substances found in plants) and xenoestrogens (chemical pollutants that mimic E2 estrogen in the body). Watch out for xenoestrogens in body care products, makeup and cleaning supplies. Even dryer sheets contains these crazy estrogen mimicking chemicals that hijack your hormones.

The E2 hormone's primary function is to regulate ovulation in a woman's reproductive years. During menopause E2 levels decrease as the ovaries don't produce any more eggs. We have over 300 estrogen receptor sites in the body and this dominating hormone plays a role in over 400 bodily functions. Many of these functions include mood, energy production, muscle strength, intestinal function, libido, brain function, and bone density. So you can see how things can get a little sideways if your estrogen levels are either too high or too low. E2 helps the body absorb minerals, decreases LDL cholesterol, increases HDL cholesterol and balances triglycerides, which reduce your risk of heart disease. If E2 levels are too high, you have an increased risk of uterine and breast cancers. When E2 levels are too low, which is common in menopause, you can be at risk for difficulties with sleep, fatigue, memory issues, depression, and increased risk of blood clots.

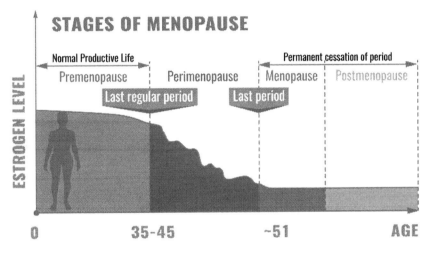

E1 is the main form of estrogen produced as you enter menopause. The ovaries ask the liver, fat cells, and adrenal glands to assist in the production of E1. During a woman's reproductive years the body converts E1 to E2, but after menopause, this conversion ceases. If your liver is sluggish and your adrenals have been stressed, it makes having a lower E2 level even more challenging.

E3 is a milder form of estrogen and its primary function is to protect the intestinal tract, vaginal lining, and breasts. Studies show that vegetarian women have higher levels of E3 and lower rates of breast cancer, playing an anti-carcinogenic role. Note: Taking synthetic hormone replacement therapies can put you at risk for breast cancer and heart disease. This is where the estrogenic effects of essential oils come into play. A few oils that I love to help balance estrogen in the body are Clary Sage, Geranium and Rose. These three powerhouse oils have been used for centuries to support women throughout their reproductive lives into their wisdom years.

Here is a list of the signs and symptoms of low and high estrogen. Now you might wonder why would I list high estrogen with menopause. Don't estrogen levels fall in menopause? Great question! It's true estrogen levels fall in menopause but all of the xenoestrogens I mentioned earlier are found in plastics and chemicals we are exposed to daily through body care products, make-up, perfumes and cleaning products. Even dryer sheets have hidden toxins in them. These xenoestrogens can keep those estrogen levels dangerously high. The Environmental Work Group (www.ewg.org) has a great list of hormone disrupting xenoestrogens. Check it out to learn more.

Take a look at these lists and make some notes on what you think your estrogen levels might be showing you. You can use your findings to start putting the puzzle pieces together. The essential oil remedies that work best for managing estrogen include lavender, clary sage, rosemary and fennel. For more information go to the Quick Reference Guides in Part 3.

Signs of Low Estrogen

- ☐ Achy Joints
- ☐ Anxiety
- ☐ Brain fog
- ☐ Depression
- ☐ Dry Eyes and/or Skin
- ☐ Leaky or Overactive Bladder
- ☐ Low Sex Drive
- ☐ Night Sweats/Hot Flashes
- ☐ Osteoporosis
- ☐ Overly Emotional
- ☐ Painful Sex
- ☐ Saggy/Shrinking Breasts
- ☐ Saggy or Thinning Skin
- ☐ Sleep Issues
- ☐ Vaginal Dryness
- ☐ Weight Gain as Belly Fat

Signs of High Estrogen

- ☐ Anxiety
- ☐ Bloating
- ☐ Breast Tenderness
- ☐ Cellulite
- ☐ Depression
- ☐ Endometriosis

- ☐ Fibroids (breast/ovary)
- ☐ Gallbladder Issues
- ☐ Headaches/Migraines
- ☐ Heavy Periods/Painful Periods
- ☐ Irritability
- ☐ Mood Swings
- ☐ PMS
- ☐ Postmenopausal Bleeding
- ☐ Sleep Issues
- ☐ Varicose Veins
- ☐ Water Retention
- ☐ Weight Gain in Hips

Understanding Progesterone

Progesterone is produced primarily by the ovaries, both before and after menopause. It's also produced by the brain and peripheral nerves. So if you have low progesterone, that's sometimes where that irritation comes from. It also accounts for itchy restless legs. We don't get excessively high levels of progesterone during peri-menopause or menopause like you do in your reproductive years. Therefore progesterone dominance is rare and why I've only included the signs of low progesterone. Progesterone is all about relaxing the smooth muscles of the body. So if we have low levels of progesterone, that can lead to levels of tension on both a physical and a mental level. Progesterone is made from cholesterol, so we need to make sure that in addition to using progesterone friendly essential oils, you are taking in healthy fats and oils in order to produce progesterone. What the body is always

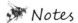

striving for is balance, particularly between estrogen and progesterone. We want these two instruments in the orchestra to be in harmony and to dance with each other in a very balanced way.

Remember progesterone affects brain function and promotes a feeling of calmness. It relaxes the smooth muscle of the intestines and other smooth muscles, particularly your heart vessels, and can help manage pain tolerance. Without enough progesterone the body can be left feeling in a state of tension and restriction.

The essential oils that I have found useful for aiding in progesterone balance include bergamot, clary sage, peppermint, thyme, sandalwood, lavender and german chamomile. Take a look at the list of signs for low progesterone and make some notes. To learn more refer to the Quick Reference Guides in Part 3.

Signs of Low Progesterone

- ☐ Anxiety
- ☐ Bloating
- ☐ Dry skin
- ☐ Fibrous Cysts (breast, ovarian or endometriosis)
- ☐ Frequent Headaches
- ☐ Heavy Painful Periods
- ☐ Hot Flashes
- ☐ Irregular Periods
- ☐ Irritability

☐ Itchy Skin Especially at Night

☐ Painful or Swollen Breasts

☐ Restless Legs

☐ Saggy Skin

☐ Water Retention

Understanding Cortisol

The truth is that in peri-menopause and menopause, the single most important hormone to be concerned about is not estrogen or progesterone, but cortisol. The levels of this hormone fluctuate up and down throughout a twenty-four hour period. When it becomes imbalanced it tends to stay elevated too long creating a domino effect on insulin, and thyroid.

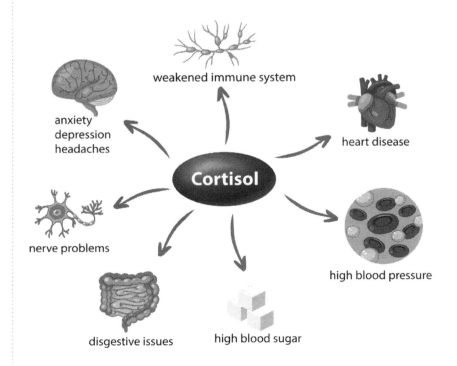

Your adrenal glands, those walnut-sized organs that sit on top of your kidneys, produce cortisol and adrenaline. A stress hormone, cortisol is designed to be used by the body in situations of acute stress to help you deal with physical danger quickly. Imagine yourself driving down the road and a deer jumps out in front of your vehicle. You swerve to miss it. Cortisol and adrenaline are activated. Cortisol also temporarily activates the immune system in case of danger, as if hitting the deer in the road has caused you physical harm or a bacteria or virus that has entered your system. It sets off an inflammatory response in which white blood cells get together to isolate the germs before attacking them. This reaction happens very quickly via the sympathetic nervous system. The problem is, that if the cortisol and its partner, epinephrine (adrenaline), don't leave the scene of the accident quickly and linger for days or even weeks or months, they have the opposite effect of lowering your immunity and energy, leaving you depleted, weak and vulnerable. At this point it begins to destroy cell membranes. This destruction results in inflammation and conditions such as leaky gut and memory issues.

Chronic fear, anger, sadness, and resentment keep stress hormones in your system too long, breaking down your immunity, thinning your skin and bones, causing weight gain, and setting the stage for poor health— including depression, cancer, and heart disease. Estrogen and progesterone get much more coverage than cortisol and adrenaline do. In my opinion cortisol and adrenaline are more likely to adversely affect your health than estrogen or progesterone.

With your ovaries now slowly decreasing their hormonal output, your adrenal glands take over some of the work of generating progesterone, along with estrogen, testosterone

Notes

and DHEA, which serves as a building block for the other hormones. But if your adrenal glands are overproducing cortisol and adrenaline, they will become very exhausted trying to keep up. They will be in survival mode and that means they won't be able to manage hormone production or the responsibilities of metabolism. They will only be focused on stress hormones and survival mode. Years ago I was really stuck in this stress loop and didn't know how to break the cycle. Through the use of essential oils, meditation and changes in my eating habits I managed to get to the other side to find balance.

When your hormones are out of balance due to hijacked cortisol, you feel the effects. You get cravings for sugar especially in the late afternoon. If you reach for a candy bar rather than taking a short walk and a drink of water to help your body break down the cortisol, you'll stimulate the adrenal glands further, causing them to release even more cortisol, which will spike your blood sugar levels. Most importantly, cortisol levels are effected by stress, blood sugar, emotions and exercise frequency. Cortisol spikes when you consume alcohol and sugar, tipping insulin out of balance as a result.

Using essential oils to reduce stress, manage cravings, balance blood sugar and improve your mental health makes the task easier to manage. Managing stress levels and getting restful sleep are two of the keys to managing cortisol. Adaptogenic essential oils can help to bring cortisol levels back to normal. Essential oils that I like to have handy each day to manage cortisol are bergamot, holy basil, pink grapefruit, frankincense, vetiver and myrrh. Use the list below and take some notes if you think you might have some issues with cortisol. See the Quick Reference Guide in Part 3 of this book to learn more.

Signs of High Cortisol

- ☐ Brain Fog
- ☐ Cry Easily
- ☐ Discolored Stretch Marks on Your Back or Belly
- ☐ Excess Belly Fat
- ☐ Experience Acid Reflux, GERD or Indigestion
- ☐ Feeling Uneasy, Moody or Shaky when Hungry
- ☐ Frequent Colds and Flu
- ☐ Get Stressed Easily
- ☐ Hair Loss
- ☐ Heart Palpitations
- ☐ Osteoporosis or Osteopenia
- ☐ Skin Issues
- ☐ Sleep Difficulties
- ☐ Struggle to be Calm, Cool and Collected
- ☐ Sugar Cravings Even After a Meal
- ☐ Tired Yet Wired
- ☐ Water Retention

Signs of Low Cortisol

- ☐ Afternoon Energy Slump
- ☐ Decreased Tolerance for Stress
- ☐ Depression
- ☐ Difficulty Making Decisions
- ☐ Dizzy Upon Standing

- ☐ Emotionally Fragile and Cry Easily
- ☐ Feelings of Being Overwhelmed
- ☐ Frequent Negative Feelings
- ☐ Hard to Get up in the Morning
- ☐ Lowered Ability to Fight Infection
- ☐ Low Blood Pressure
- ☐ Low Sex Drive
- ☐ Low or Unstable Blood Sugar
- ☐ Salt Cravings
- ☐ Severe Fatigue or Burnout

Understanding Insulin

Insulin is made by the pancreas. Remember the pancreas is one of the organs that makes up the endocrine system although most doctors never describe it this way. Its function is to remove sugar from the blood and take it to your cells. Insulin is the hormone that tells our cells to pick up glucose from the bloodstream. It is also the major energy storage hormone in the body. It tells our cells to store energy, either as glycogen or fat. It also determines where your fat is stored. When cortisol is elevated it triggers insulin to store more fat, especially around your waist, hips and thighs. Yikes! At this point we lose our feminine curves and take on an apple or pear shaped body.

Excess sugar is stored in fat cells. When this happens it is called hyperinsulinemia. This condition is a major contributor of inflammation in the body. If insulin remains too high, insulin receptors on the cells lose their ability to respond to high blood sugar. This creates insulin resistance, leading to type 2 diabetes. Body fat is loaded with insulin receptors. The more body fat you have, the more insulin it takes to get the blood sugar into your cells. Because insulin is a storage hormone, the higher its levels, the harder it is for the body to release it as fuel. Insulin actually locks the fat in place.

High insulin levels not only raise cortisol levels but also triggers high blood pressure and thickening of the walls of the blood vessels, a condition known as arteriosclerosis. It increases water retention in the body and contributes to depression. Elevated insulin interferes with the conversion of T-4 to T-3 and leads to hypothyroidism.

When insulin levels rise, the orchestra of hormones is definitely playing off key. Estrogen loses its able to metabolize properly and HDL cholesterol is affected. In short, when insulin is elevated it causes a chain reaction of hormone imbalances and therefore increased symptoms, especially headaches, PMS, hot flashes and night sweats. This perfect storm also creates an environment in the body to invite ovarian and breast cysts and an increase in your chances of cancer. Studies have shown that maintaining healthy insulin levels helps prevent breast cancer. The bottom line is to manage your insulin levels carefully to stave off this host of conditions.

Some of the most helpful essential oils for balancing insulin include cinnamon, clary sage, myrrh, sweet orange and ylang ylang. Use the list below to take some notes if you think you might have some issues with insulin. See the Quick Reference Guide in Part 3 of this book to learn more.

Signs of High Insulin
(Insulin Resistance)

☐ Cardiovascular Issues

☐ Cellulite

☐ Constant Cravings for Sweets and Carbs

☐ Extreme Thirst or Hunger

☐ Fasting Glucose Level Higher than 90mg/dL

☐ Fatigue Throughout the Day

☐ Feeling Hungry After a Meal

☐ Frequent or Increased Urination

☐ Hair Growth on Upper Lip, Chin or Nipples

☐ Hemoglobin A1c Higher than 5.4

☐ High LDL Cholesterol or High Triglycerides

☐ High Blood Pressures

☐ Irregular Periods

☐ Tingling Sensations in Hands and Feet

☐ Tired After a Meal

☐ Vision Changes or Cataracts

☐ Weight Gain

Understanding Thyroid

In peri-menopause and menopause the most common imbalance in the thyroid is known as hypothyroidism or low thyroid. An estimated 20 million Americans have some form of thyroid disease. Up to 60 percent of those with thyroid disease are unaware of their condition. Women are five to eight times more likely than men to have thyroid problems.

One woman in eight will develop a thyroid disorder during her lifetime. Hypothyroidism is most common in middle aged women. Right about the time you are going through peri-menopause and menopause. It's no coincidence.

In a 2011 study, researchers examined the role that estrogen levels have on thyroid receptors. Thyroid receptors are the molecules that allow thyroid hormones to enter cells. Researchers found that estrogen levels might affect thyroid function and lead to thyroid disorders. More research is needed to better understand the relationship between these two hormones. Initial results point to estrogen having a role in the thyroid's ability to function.

The thyroid is that butterfly shaped gland at the base of your throat. It is a hormone-producing gland that regulates the body's metabolism—the rate at which the body produces energy from nutrients and oxygen—and affects critical body functions, such as energy level and heart rate. Although the thyroid gland is relatively small, it produces a hormone that influences every cell, tissue and organ in the body. I like to think of it as the gas pedal on your car. If it isn't getting enough gas it will slowly chug along and eventually stall out. A thyroid that isn't working properly can lead to a host of conditions. Conventional blood tests don't always reveal problems with this gland because most doctors only test your TSH levels. A good test will include your TPO antibodies. That is a better indicator of what is really going on.

Certain common drugs suppress thyroid activity including aspirin, corticosteroids and anticoagulants. Even fluoride and chlorine in drinking water can effect thyroid function. That's why it's important to filter your drinking water. I use the Berkey filter.

Notes

Here is how the body produces thyroid hormone. The hypothalamus in the brain is the master regulator for the body's hormones. When the hypothalamus detects the need for thyroid hormones, it produces TRH. The TRH goes to the pituitary gland and produces TSH. Then TSH makes its way through the blood to bind to the receptor sites in the thyroid. This stimulates the thyroid to produce T4 and T3. The T3 is more active. T4 is more of a storage hormone. T4 is converted to T3 in peripheral tissues (20% conversion by the liver and 20% conversion by the intestines). If the liver is congested it may not be converting T4 to T3 properly. If the intestinal tract is inflamed or you have leaky gut or celiac disease it may also have difficulty converting T4 to T3 and compromise the thyroid function. It's just another section of the hormonal orchestra that needs to be fine tuned.

As the primary regulator of metabolism and fuel burning, the thyroid monitors fat. When thyroid output is low the body tends to store fat instead of burn it. Thus the weight gain despite all of our efforts to eat healthy and exercise. This in turn causes other hormones to shift out of balance. If thyroid imbalance continues it can develop into Hashimoto's disease which is an autoimmune disorder. As a health coach I believe that in addition to using essential oils, maintaining a diet that is free of alcohol, caffeine, grains, dairy and sugar can help all the body systems resolve thyroid issues.

Thyroid supporting oils I've had good results with include clove, myrrh, lemongrass and frankincense. Use the list below to take some notes if you think you might have some issues with thyroid. See the Quick Reference Guide in Part 3 of this book to learn more.

Signs of Low Thyroid

- ☐ Anxiety
- ☐ Brain Fog
- ☐ Brittle Nails and Hair
- ☐ Compromised Immune System
- ☐ Constipation
- ☐ Depression
- ☐ Dry Skin
- ☐ Enlarged Thyroid
- ☐ Experience Hives
- ☐ Frequently Tired
- ☐ Hair Loss of Eyebrows or Eyelashes
- ☐ Hair Loss on Head
- ☐ High LDL Cholesterol
- ☐ Indentations on the Sides of Your Tongue
- ☐ Lethargy
- ☐ Low Sex Drive
- ☐ Painful Achy Muscles and Joints
- ☐ Tingling in Feet and Hands
- ☐ Weight Gain Despite Diet and Exercise

Some other hormones worth mentioning that play a part in the hormonal orchestra are leptin, cholesterol and oxytocin.

Understanding Leptin

When I discovered how the hormone leptin works in the body I thought I had found the holy grail. This little known hormone was only discovered by scientists in 1994. It intricately interlaces in the endocrine system with cortisol and insulin. It is the appetite hormone, working with ghrelin to balance hunger and satiation. It helps control your metabolism. Leptin is also responsible for regulating blood pressure and heart rate, activating immune cells and regulating synthesis of the thyroid hormones. When this hormone is in balance it decreases glucose, working with insulin to balance blood sugar. In part it helps regulate your menstrual cycle and has an effect on healthy bone mass.

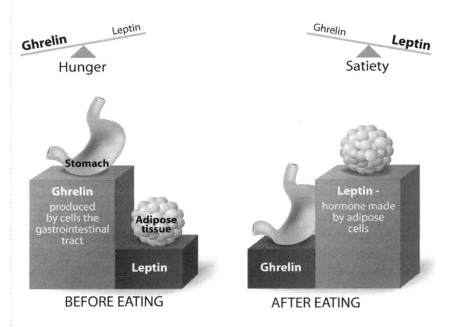

When leptin is out of balance, the symptoms can mimic insulin resistance. Leptin becomes elevated when stress levels go up. This keeps you in a state of constant hunger that is never satisfied. Leptin is controlled by insulin. However, regular exercise and restful sleep can bring this hormone back into balance.

Some of the best essential oils to balance leptin are pink grapefruit, lemon, sweet orange and peppermint.

Understanding Cholesterol

Here is another hormones that no one ever tells you about. We are taught that cholesterol is bad for you. Well, I'm here to show you how useful and important it is in hormone balance. The primary use of 60-80% of the cholesterol in our bodies is to make bile for the digestion of fats. The brain uses cholesterol as well. After the brain, the organs hungriest for cholesterol are our endocrine glands: adrenals and sex glands. They produce steroid hormones. The steroid hormones in the body made from cholesterol include: testosterone, progesterone, pregnenolone, androsterone, estrone, estradiol, corticosterone, aldosterone and others. Yes, these are more instruments in the hormonal orchestra that must be in tune and be in sufficient amounts to make beautiful music.

These hormones accomplish a myriad of functions in the body, from regulation of our metabolism, energy production, mineral assimilation, brain, muscle and bone formation to behavior, emotions and reproduction. In our stressful modern lives we consume a lot of these hormones, leading to a condition called "adrenal exhaustion." Cholesterol is used to make adrenal and reproductive hormones and to round up toxins in the body.

Saturated fats and cholesterol create the membrane of the cells and make them firm—without them the cells would become fluid and flabby. Cholesterol and saturated fats firm up and reinforce the tissues in the body such as our blood vessels, particularly those that have to withstand the high pressure of the blood flow.

Actually, cholesterol levels below 175 can put you at risk for depression, infertility, increased cancer risks and an increased chance of a heart attack. I see growing numbers of people with memory loss who have been taking cholesterol-lowering medications over a long period of time. We need cholesterol. Low levels of cholesterol have been linked to adrenal fatigue, thyroid issues and many hormone imbalances.

Early signs of insulin resistance are reflected in low HDL cholesterol levels. These are the good cholesterol and we need them to help in the harmonious hormone balance. If you reach full blown metabolic syndrome your cholesterol swings the other direction to being very high.

Omega 3 fatty acids help to lower triglycerides and fiber can benefit cholesterol balance as well. Including these good fats in your diet is critical. Processed foods and artificial fats decrease HDL (good cholesterol) and increase LDL (bad cholesterol). Since cholesterol interfaces with so many hormones in the body it makes sense that the essential oils that support estrogen, progesterone and cortisol would be in order. The oils that I like to use also support the cardiovascular system.

Topping the list are clary sage, basil, lemongrass, bergamot and rosemary essential oils.

Understanding Oxytocin

Oxytocin is the love and bonding hormone. It is a major conductor in the hormone family. It's the "feel good" hormone. It gives us a sense of connection, creates pleasure, joy and harmony. It increases our tolerance for pain. It's how a woman can go through the pains of labor and delivery and the minute she holds that baby in her arms the oxytocin flows through her system filling her with love and connection with her child. People with pets have higher levels of oxytocin than those who don't. It is important to find things during this menopausal transition that bring you joy and turn on this love and bonding hormone. This is a time to develop meaningful authentic friendships with other women traveling this same road.

Essential oils that stimulate the brain to send out oxytocin are rose, sandalwood and jasmine.

Three conditions that plague millions of women during peri-menopause and menopause are hot flashes, PMS and weight gain. I feel it's important to give these subjects a bit more explanation.

Hot Flashes & Night Sweats Explained

Nearly every woman over the age of 40 that I have talked to, has had a hot flash. It is estimated that two-thirds to three-quarters of all American women in mid-life experience hot flashes. They can last anywhere from a few months to up to 10 years and can significantly affect a woman's quality of life. Night sweats, in particular, can erode your overall health because they disrupt sleep, which can lead to mental and physical concerns. Here is the anatomy behind a hot flash.

The sequence of events that causes a hot flash.

1. Estrogen levels decrease in peri-menopause and menopause, signaling the hypothalamus to pull the alarm and tell the body it's too hot.

2. You begin to sweat because that's how the body cools off.

3. Blood vessels dilate to allow the blood to come to the surface of your skin. Your skin temperature rises and you feel hot.

4. Your heart pumps blood faster, in order to circulate blood and cool you off. This can make you feel dizzy, anxious, claustrophobic and hot.

5. As the blood rushes to the surface of your skin, your face, chest and neck get red and blotchy.

6. You begin to sweat in order to get rid of the excess heat.

7. After about five minutes, you're a hot sweaty mess, then you begin to cool off, and your brain believes your temperature has regulated. The hot flash is over.

Anatomy of a Hot Flash

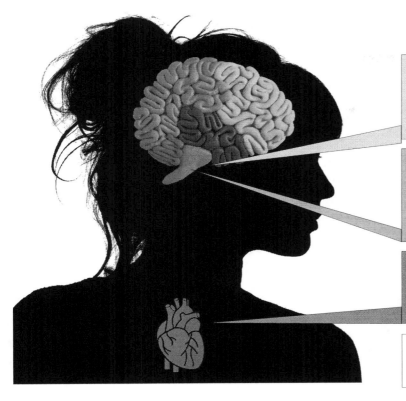

#1 - Decreasing estrogen has effects on the hypothalamus that confuse it with inaccurate messages that the body is too hot.

#2 - The brain responds by sending out a red alert to the heart, blood vessels and nervous system that the body needs to be cooled off.

#3 - The heart pumps faster and blood vessels open up to circulate more blood and activate the sweat glands.

#4 - You're having a hot flash!

Symptoms you may experience associated with hot flashes can include:

- flushing and skin blotchiness

- chills and shivering

- anxiety

- tingling, crawling skin sensation (formication)

- increased heart rate and/or palpitations

- weakness

- feeling trapped or suffocated

Anxiety, fear and emotional stress can increase the chanc-

🐝 Notes

es of having hot flashes and night sweats. Scientific research confirms that stress is a major hot flash trigger. Studies show that women who are depressed, in low socioeconomic positions, or who were abused or neglected in early life have more frequent hot flashes. Relaxation techniques, meditation, hypnosis, counseling and cognitive-behavioral training have been shown to help.

Many types of stress can lead to increased levels of stress hormones, including insulin resistance and smoking. If the incidence of hot flashes increase when your body is under stress and tension it points to estrogen, progesterone, cortisol and insulin playing a role here as well.

Essential oils that are beneficial in calming hot flashes and night sweats include clary sage, cypress, peppermint and geranium.

 Tip:

80-90% of women in our culture experience hot flashes & night sweats

PMS Unraveled

We have probably all experienced that nagging monthly headache, backache, and bite-your-head-off responses to those around us. I know you just want to shut the world out or self-medicate with a pan of brownies or raw cookie dough. Believe me, I've been there! I also want you to know that this is NOT NORMAL. It can however be relieved and even eliminated over time using essential oils, herbs, and dietary changes.

PMS, or premenstrual syndrome, encompasses a group of symptoms that often affect women in the days prior to and up to the beginning of their menstrual flow. It can have an effect on women who are just starting their menarche, usually during adolescent years, and symptoms can continue well into menopause. PMS typically affects women between their 20's and 40's most significantly. PMS essentially occurs when there is decreased progesterone and increased estrogen in your body.

Estrogen Dominance

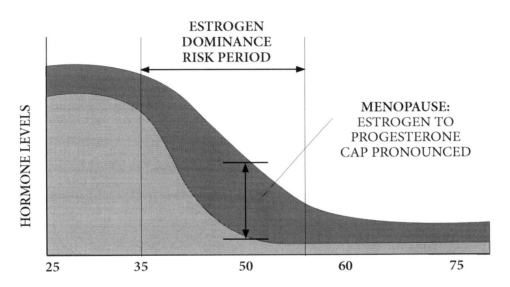

Symptoms of PMS include emotional distress, mood swings, depression, aggression, anxiety, stress, and mental state alteration. Physical symptoms include fatigue, bloating, cramps, breast tenderness, low back pain, fluid retention, and headaches. PMS affects some women more adversely than others. According to Dr. Henry G. Beiler, who wrote *Food Is Your Best Medicine,* there are three lines of defense in the body: the gastrointestinal system, which allows you to digest food and absorb nutrients; the hepatic system, or liver, that filters toxins from the blood and intestines; and the endocrine system, which are the hormones that regulate menstrual cycles and hormone levels in the body throughout the month. Your hormones communicate with the microbiome of your gut and your immune system.

These systems work intricately with each other. When any of these lines of defense are compromised, the rest of the body suffers. Here is how your body gets "set-up" to have the perfect PMS storm:

1. If you are eating food that is not nutrient dense or is processed, you can't absorb the correct nutrients and toxins can begin to build up in your digestive system. This could prompt yeast and candida overgrowth or intestinal bacteria that is harmful. This is the first breakdown in the body's defense system.

2. The liver is forced to take on a heavier load to remove excess toxin through the blood. It gets angry at having this extra responsibility and responds by initiating hot flashes, night sweats or a snappy temper.

3. The endocrine system has been getting poor communication from both the digestive system and the liver and becomes confused on how to respond. It begins to misfire as the toxic load is shifted to the last detox organ–the uterus. This hormonal response is the origin of PMS symptoms. In PMS, the uterus is used as an organ of elimination of toxins in the blood such as excess estrogen. The cramps, discomforts, and congestion associated with PMS are the result of toxins accumulating in the pelvic region prior to menses. In menopausal women who are no longer having a regular period it becomes even more important to keep the digestive system and liver in tip top shape.

4. Edema, or fluid retention, is created by the inability of the kidneys to handle these toxins. Pain and headaches are due to the irritating effects toxins. Finally, heavy menstrual flow, which results in weakness, anxiety, and anemia, is caused by the body trying to rid itself of as much toxic material as possible.

Thus, all PMS symptoms are related to a general toxicity of the blood. Over time these same toxins irritate the female organs sufficiently to cause cysts, fibroids, and other chronic reproductive problems.

I like to take a comprehensive approach to PMS and imbalances in the body using food, herbs, and essential oils.

Some of the essential oils that I have found helpful in easing PMS are ylang ylang, bergamot, geranium, fennel and palmarosa.

"Angela does a fantastic job listening and understanding what is going on with me/my body. She explains what might be at play and what oils would be helpful and why. The combinations of oils are always helpful and get me back on track."

~ Venus

Managing Healthy Weight through Menopause

Maintaining a healthy body weight is often a challenge for women, especially as you get older. Your metabolism isn't what it used to be. Maybe you have a stressful job or family demands that don't allow you the time to prepare healthy meals or even manage some self care. Perhaps your hormones are imbalanced and you find yourself in a daily battle with the bathroom scales. If any of these scenarios sound familiar it's time to introduce you to the aromatic world of essential oils and their role in helping you reach your healthy weight goals, balance key hormones, and uplift your mood. When cortisol is elevated with stress then insulin gets disrupted. Soon the thyroid is involved and metabolism hits a wall.

Some of you may be wondering how an essential oil can do all of that. Believe me, I was once skeptical about this as well until I began using aromatherapy to help curb sugar cravings, which was something I battled with for years. I discovered that not only did my cravings diminish but my mood increased and I found myself much more relaxed and able to make better choices toward a more healthy lifestyle and way of eating.

How essential oils can help with weight loss:

- curb appetite

- increase metabolism

- burn fat

- improve digestion

- reduce sugar and carb cravings

- detoxify the body

- alkalize and balance

- increase positive mood

Dieting alone often produces temporary results, and if the body feels that it's being "starved" then the reverse can happen, creating "diet-induced weight gain." This is the exact opposite effect you were going for and can leave you feeling lost and depressed and reaching for that candy bar you had stashed away for emergencies.

I've always been a big fan bringing some solid strategies together that include portion control, eating fresh foods, and zero tolerance for processed foods as part of a healthy weight loss plan. Having the right mindset to accomplish your weight goals is also a key to success. To support a well-rounded wellness plan there are several key essential oils to bring onboard. These include pink grapefruit, lemon, sweet orange, fennel and geranium.

Pink Grapefruit – In research studies, Pink Grapefruit oil helps initiate the hormone leptin or satiation hormone. This makes you feel full sooner and satisfied with eating less. Add this to a diffuser during the day to aid in healthy weight loss.

Lemon – This oil is a diuretic and supports the circulatory and lymphatic systems. It brings focus and clarity to your intentions to lose weight and uplifts mood by supporting the nervous system. Lemon is also a mild detoxifier as well.

Sweet Orange – This oil is used as a digestive tonic and lymphatic stimulant to help detoxify the body. It helps to circulate stagnant energy when it accumulates in the liver, stomach, and intestines. It is one of the best oils for the digestive system.

Fennel – This oil plays is stellar role when it comes to stimulating digestion. It gives you a sense of fullness and helps avoid overeating. It has the ability to increase metabolism.

Geranium – As a balancing oil it has the ability to reduce cravings for sugar and carbs. Just rub this oil on the bottoms of your feet morning and night to reduce cravings.

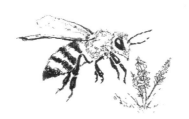

PART 3

Quick Reference Guides

Hormone Symptom Mapper

Symptom	Low Estrogen	High Estrogen	Low Progesterone	High Cortisol	Low Cortisol	High Insulin	Low Thyroid
Achy joints/muscles	X						X
Anxiety	X	X	X				X
Brain Fog	X			X			
Breast Tenderness		X	X				
Bloating		X	X				
Cellulite		X					
Cravings Sugar/Salt				X Sugar	X Salt	X Sugar	
Depression	X	X					X
Dry, Itchy Skin/Eyes	X		X	X			X
Easily Stressed				X	X		
Emotionally Sensitive	X			X	X		
Fatigue					X	X	X
Frequently Sick					X		X

Symptom	Low Estrogen	High Estrogen	Low Progesterone	High Cortisol	Low Cortisol	High Insulin	Low Thyroid
Fibroids (breast ovary)		X	X				
Hair Loss				X			
Headaches		X	X				
Heart Palpitations				X			
High Cholesterol						X	X
Hot Flashes	X		X				
Irritability		X	X				
Low Sex Drive	X				X		X
Mood Swings		X		X			
Osteoporosis	X			X			
Painful Irregular Periods		X	X			X	
Painful Sex/Vaginal Dryness	X						
Post-menopausal Bleeding		X					
Saggy Skin/Breasts	X		X				
Sleep Issues	X	X		X			
Unstable or High Blood Sugar				X	X	X	
Weight Gain	X	X	X	X		X	X
Water Retention		X	X	X			

Essential Oil Remedy Mapper

Essential Oil	Low Estrogen	High Estrogen	Low Progesterone	High Cortisol	Low Cortisol	High Insulin	Low Thyroid
Atlas Cedarwood	X		X	X			X
Bergamot		X	X	X	X	X	
Black Spruce	X	X	X	X			X
Blue Tansy				X	X		
Cinnamon bark/leaf	X	X		X	X	X	X
Clary Sage	X	X	X			X	
Clove	X				X		X
Cypress	X	X	X	X		X	X
Eucalyptus	X			X	X	X	X
Fennel	X	X		X		X	X
Frankincense	X		X	X			X
Geranium	X	X	X	X		X	X
German Chamomile	X	X	X	X			X
Ginger	X	X	X				X
Green Myrtle	X	X		X		X	
Holy Basil				X	X	X	X
Jasmine	X	X			X		X
Lavender	X	X	X	X	X	X	X
Lemon	X	X	X	X	X	X	X
Lemongrass		X		X		X	X
Linden Blossom	X	X	X	X			
Mandarin		X		X	X		
May Chang	X		X	X	X		X
Melissa (Lemon Balm)	X	X	X	X		X	X
Myrrh	X		X	X		X	X

Essential Oil	Low Estrogen	High Estrogen	Low Progesterone	High Cortisol	Low Cortisol	High Insulin	Low Thyroid
Neroli	X	X		X			
Nutmeg	X		X	X	X		X
Oregano	X		X	X	X	X	X
Palmarosa	X	X	X	X			X
Patchouli	X	X		X	X		X
Peppermint	X		X	X	X	X	X
Pine Needle	X	X	X	X			X
Pink Grapefruit	X	X	X	X	X	X	X
Roman Chamomile		X	X		X		X
Rose Otto	X	X	X	X		X	
Rosemary	X	X	X	X	X	X	X
Sandalwood	X	X	X		X		X
Sweet Marjoram	X	X	X	X			
Sweet Orange	X	X		X		X	X
Tea Tree	X			X	X	X	X
Thyme	X	X	X		X		X
Vetiver	X	X		X	X		X
Ylang Ylang	X	X		X	X	X	X

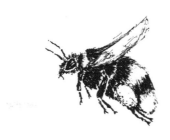

PART 4

100 Essential Oil Recipes

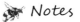

Measurement Key
1/2 oz. = 1 Tablespoon
1 oz. = 2 Tablespoons

Improve Your Mood

The top essential oils for improving mood are:

- Bergamot

- Pink Grapefruit

- Lemon

- Green Mandarin

- Sweet Orange

- Ylang Ylang

Woman's Balance Bath Soak Blend

A therapeutic blend to uplift your mood and balance hormones.

Materials:

small glass mixing bowl

Ingredients:

1 cup epsom salts or magnesium flakes

1 teaspoon sweet almond oil

3 drops Clary Sage *(Salvia sclarea)*

1 drop Frankincense *(Boswelli carterii)*

3 drops Lavender *(Lavandula angustifolia)*

1 drop Red Mandarin *(Citrus reticulata)*

1 drop Sweet Orange *(Citrus sinensis)*

1 drop Ylang Ylang *(Cananga odorata)*

Directions:

Mix essential oils and sweet almond oil then add to bath salts. Soak for 20-30 minutes. Take some time to be mindful of actually feeling your body relax. Notice how you feel after you soak.

Menopause Wellbeing Diffuser Blend

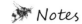

Materials:

    5 ml amber bottle

Ingredients:

    20 drops Neroli *(Citrus aurantium)*

    35 drops Lavender *(Lavandula angustifolia)*

    35 drops Bergamot *(Citrus bergamia)*

    10 drops Patchouli *(Pogostemon cablin)*

Directions:

Mix all oils in 5 ml bottle, place lid on and shake well to blend. Use several drops in a diffuser for calming, balancing and uplifting feelings.

Depression Free Aroma Inhaler

Materials:

    blank inhaler

    small glass mixing bowl

Ingredients:

    5 drops Pink Grapefruit *(Citrus paradisi)*

    3 drops Lemon *(Citrus limon)*

    3 drops Bergamot *(Citrus bergamia)*

    1 drop Neroli *(Citrus aurantium)*

Directions:

Mix oils together and dip cotton wick into the mixture and let it absorb the oil blend. Place wick inside the blank inhaler and cap. Remove lid and place in nostril (closing off other nostril) and take several slow deep breaths. Repeat in other nostril. Use as often as needed for stress.

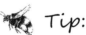 Tip:

80-90% of women in our culture experience hot flashes & night sweats

Anxiety Free Aroma Inhaler

This is my personal favorite blend. It calms my mind and I love it as an inhaler to have handy with me at all times.

Materials:
    blank inhaler
    small glass mixing bowl

Ingredients:
    5 drops Bergamot *(Citrus bergamia)*
    3 drops Lavender *(Lavandula angustifolia)*
    1 drop Roman Chamomile *(Chamaemelum nobilis)*
    1 drop Ylang Ylang *(Cananga odorata)*

Directions:

Mix oils together and pour onto cotton wick and put inside the blank inhaler. Place cap on and label. Remove lid and place in nostril (closing off other nostril) and take several deep breaths. Repeat in other nostril. Use as often as needed for anxiety relief.

"When I first tried essential oils for anxiety I didn't really think they would work but after only a few days of using an inhaler my husband said I was like a different person, in a good way! Now I don't freak out in traffic or turn down social gatherings. What a sense of freedom."
                                                                    ~Margie

Anxiety Relief Roll-On

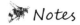

Materials:

1/3 oz. roll-on bottle

Ingredients:

1/3 oz. jojoba oil

3 drops Bergamot *(Citrus bergamia)*

3 drops Kaffir Lime *(Citrus hystrix)*

3 drops Sweet Orange *(Citrus sinensis)*

2 drops Sandalwood *(Santalum album)*

1 drop Vetiver *(Vetiveria zizanoides)*

Directions:

Add essential oils to roll-on ball bottle. Mix well. Add the jojoba oil, put roller ball and lid on and shake well. Apply to your wrists, chest, neck and bottom of feet as often as needed to relieve anxiety.

Anxiety Diffuser Blend

Materials:

5ml amber bottle

Ingredients:

30 drops Clary Sage *(Salvia sclarea)*

20 drops Bergamot *(Citrus bergamia)*

15 drops Geranium *(Pelargonium roseum x asperum)*

10 drops Roman Chamomile *(Chamaemelum nobilis)*

15 drops Sweet Marjoram *(Origanum marjorana)*

10 drops Ylang Ylang *(Cananga odorata)*

Directions:

Mix all essential oils and place in a 5ml amber bottle. Place several drops in a diffuser to help reduce anxiety.

Anxiety Release Spritzer

Materials:

2 oz. amber glass bottle with spritzer top

Ingredients:

1.5 oz organic witch hazel

2 droppers distress remedy homeopathic

8 drops Lavender *(Lavandula angustifolia)*

5 drops Clary Sage *(Salvia sclarea)*

7 drops Green Mandarin *(Citrus reticulata var. mandarine)*

4 drops Roman Chamomile *(Chamaemelum nobilis)*

4 drops Holy Basil *(Ocimum sanctum)*

2 drops Patchouli *(Pogostemon cablin)*

Directions:

Mix all essential oils together and add distress remedy homeopathic and mix well. Add mixture to glass bottle and fill with Witch Hazel. Place spray top on and shake well. Spritz over head and shoulders avoiding eye area several times a day to manage feelings of anxiety.

 Tip:

Fluctuations in estrogen and progesterone levels can cause anxiety and panic attacks

Emotional Calm Aroma Inhaler

Brings forth a deep sense of calm

Materials:
    blank Inhaler
    small glass mixing bowl

Ingredients:
    1 drop Roman Chamomile *(Chamaemelum nobilis)*
    4 drops Lavender *(Lavandula angustifolia)*
    6 drops Rosewood *(Aniba roseodora)*
    1 drop Ylang Ylang *(Cananga odorata)*

Directions:
Place essential oils on the cotton wick and insert into inhaler blank. Place cap on and label. Twist off cap and inhale whenever you feel a need for calming.

Nervous System Sedative Lotion

Effective for Calming and supporting

Materials:
    2 oz. glass jar

Ingredients:
    2 oz. organic unscented lotion
    10 drops Green Mandarin *(Citrus reticulata var. mandarine)*
    5 drops Roman Chamomile *(Chamaemelum nobilis)*
    10 drops Neroli *(Citrus aurantium)*
    5 drops Ylang Ylang *(Cananga odorata)*

Directions:
Blend essential oils and add to 2 oz of unscented lotion. Mix thoroughly. Apply to your neck, throat, and chest 3 times a day.

Notes

Antidepressant Spray

Helps to prevent and alleviate depression

Materials:

    2 oz. dark glass bottle with spritzer top

Ingredients:

    2 oz. rose hydrosol
    6 drops Bergamot *(Citrus bergamia)*
    4 drops Pink Grapefruit *(Citrus paradisi)*
    5 drops Jasmine *(Jasminum grandiflorum)*
    5 drops Kaffir Lime *(Citrus hystrix)*

Directions:

Add essential oils to 2 oz Spray bottle filled with rose hydrosol. Place   lid on and shake well. Spritz the blend above your head (with eyes closed) and breath deeply! Use as often as needed for feelings of depression.

Focus & Brain Fog Remedies

The top essential oils for focus and brain fog are:

- Eucalyptus

- Rosemary

- Peppermint

Brain Fog Buster

This spritzer really helps clear out the cobwebs and gets your memory and concentration back on track.

Materials:

    2 oz. dark glass bottle with spray top

Ingredients:

    2 oz. organic witch hazel
    5 drops Eucalyptus *(Eucalyptus radiata)*
    6 drops Rosemary *(Rosmarinus officinalis ct. verbenone)*
    6 drops Peppermint *(Mentha x Piperita)*
    9 drops May Chang *(Litsea cubeba)*
    4 drops Frankincense *(Boswelli carterii)*

Directions:

Add essential oils to 2 oz spray bottle filled with witch hazel . Place lid on and shake well. Spritz the blend above your head (with eyes closed) and breath deeply! Use as often as needed for brain fog and concentration.

Radical Focus Aroma Inhaler

Increases your ability to focus and relieves mental chatter

Materials:
    blank Inhaler
    small glass mixing bowl

Ingredients:
    2 drops Sweet Orange *(Citrus sinensis)*
    1 drop Peppermint *(Mentha X piperita)*
    7 drops Ravintsara *(Cinnamomum camphora ct. cineole)*

Directions:
Mix oils together and pour onto cotton wick and put inside the blank inhaler. Place cap on and label. Remove lid and place in nostril (closing off other nostril) and take several deep breaths. Repeat in other nostril. Use as often as needed to focus.

Concentration Blend

Materials:
    5ml amber glass bottle

Ingredients:
    40 drops Lemon *(Citrus limon)*
    30 drops Holy Basil *(Ocimum sanctum)*
    30 drops Rosemary *(Rosmarinus officinalis ct. verbenone)*

Directions:
Mix essential oils together and place in 5ml amber glass bottle. Use several drops in diffuser to enhance concentration.

Stress Management Solutions

The top essential oils for stress management are:

- Lavender
- Holy Basil
- Bergamot
- Blue Tansy
- Red Mandarin

Stress Relief Bath Soak

Let the stress of the day just melt away

Materials:
small glass mixing bowl

Ingredients:
1 cup magnesium flakes
1 teaspoon sweet almond oil
6 drops Geranium *(Pelargonium roseum x asperum)*
12 drops Lavender *(Lavandula angustifolia)*
6 drops Blue Tansy *(Tanacetum annuum)*
6 drops Ylang Ylang *(Cananga odorata)*

Directions:
Place magnesium flakes into the glass bowl. Add essential oils and sweet almond oil into the magnesium flakes and mix thoroughly. Place mixture into bath water. Soak for 20-30 minutes. Relieves stress, supports the nervous system & endocrine system.

Stress Be Gone Massage Oil

Materials:
  2 oz. dark glass bottle with dropper lid
  small glass mixing bowl

Ingredients:
  2 oz. fractionated coconut oil
  8 drops Atlas Cedarwood *(Cedrus atlantica)*
  15 drops Pink Grapefruit *(Citrus paradisi)*
  7 drops Lavender *(Lavandula angustifolia)*

Directions:
Fill the bottle with 1 oz. coconut oil then add the essential oils and shake well. Add the remaining 1 oz. coconut oil, place lid on and shake well. Use 1 dropper full to massage arms, legs, shoulders and chest or apply to bottoms of feet to reduce stress and tension.

 Tip:

When stress levels are elevated, menopause symptoms such as hot flashes, irritability and cravings increase as well.

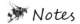

Stress Be Gone Roll-On

Materials:

1/3 oz. roll-on bottle

Ingredients:

1/3 oz. organic jojoba oil

3 drops Red Mandarin *(Citrus reticulata)*

2 drops Rose *(Rosa damascena)*

3 drops Bergamot *(Citrus bergamia)*

2 drops Ylang Ylang *(Cananga odorata)*

Directions:

Place essential oils in roll-on ball bottle and swirl to mix. Add 1/2 of the jojoba oil and swirl to mix again. Add remainder of the jojoba oil and place the roller ball and cap on and gently rock back and forth to completely mix all ingredients. Use 2-3 times a day on wrists, neck, heart space or bottoms of feet to reduce feelings of stress.

Peace And Tranquility Blend

Materials:

5ml amber bottle

Ingredients:

15 drops Roman Chamomile *(Chamaemelum nobilis)*

30 drops Melissa, Lemon Balm *(Melissa officinalis)*

25 drops Rose Otto *(Rosa damascena)*

30 drops Lavender *(Lavandula angustifolia)*

Directions:

Mix oils together and place in a 5ml bottle and use in diffuser to create a peaceful environment.

Emotional Calming Aroma Inhaler

Materials:

blank Inhaler

small glass mixing bowl

Ingredients:

1 drop Roman Chamomile *(Chamaemelum nobilis)*

4 drops Lavender *(Lavandula angustifolia)*

5 drops Rosewood *(Aniba roseodora)*

2 drops Ylang Ylang *(Cananga odorata)*

Directions:

Mix oils together and pour onto cotton wick and put inside the blank inhaler and cap. Remove lid and place in nostril (closing off other nostril) and take several deep breaths. Repeat in other nostril. Use as often as needed for calming.

 Tip:

All essential oils are adaptogenic and work to help cells manage stress and renew.

Chill Out Spritzer

Materials:

2 oz. dark glass bottle with spray top

Ingredients:

2 oz. rose hydrosol

16 drops Pink Grapefruit *(Citrus paradisi)*

2 drops Patchouli *(Pogostemon cablin)*

5 drops Rose Otto *(Rosa damascena)*

3 drops Vetiver *(Vetiveria zizanoides)*

4 drops Ylang Ylang *(Cananga odorata)*

Directions:

Combine all essential oils and mix thoroughly. Add to rose hydrosol and pour into 2 oz. glass bottle with spritzer top. Shake well before each use. Spritz over head and shoulders avoiding eyes when stress builds up and you need to chill out.

BP Ease Roll-On

This blend has a gentling effect on blood pressure while balancing hormones

Materials:

1/3 oz. roll-on bottle

Ingredients:

1/3 oz. sweet almond oil

2 drops Ylang Ylang *(Cananga odorata)*

3 drops Lemon *(Citrus limon)*

2 drops Lavender *(Lavandula angustifolia)*

2 drops Sweet Marjoram *(Origanum marjorana)*

2 drops Clary Sage *(Salvia sclarea)*

Directions:

Place all ingredients in roll-on bottle and place roller ball and lid on. Shake well to blend. Apply to wrists, neck and heart space several times a day.

"Angela's essential oil blends have eased my menopause and blood pressure issues over the past 3 years tremendously."

~Lynn

De-Stress This Mess Aroma Inhaler

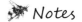

Materials:

    blank inhaler
    small glass mixing bowl

Ingredients:

    4 drops Bergamot *(Citrus bergamia)*
    2 drops Pink Grapefruit *(Citrus paradisi)*
    1 drops Frankincense *(Boswelli carterii)*
    1 drops Neroli *(Citrus aurantium)*
    2 drops Clary Sage *(Salvia sclarea)*

Directions:

Mix oils together in small bowl and dip cotton wick into the mixture and let it absorb the oil blend. Place wick inside the blank inhaler and cap. Remove lid and place in nostril (closing off other nostril) and take several slow deep breaths. Repeat in other nostril. Use as often as needed for stress.

The top essential oils for improving energy are:

- Lemon

- Peppermint

- Eucalyptus

- Pink Grapefruit

Energize Me Aroma Inhaler

Materials:
blank inhaler
small glass mixing bowl

Ingredients:
4 drops Lavender *(Lavandula angustifolia)*
2 drops Lemon *(Citrus limon)*
5 drops Sweet Orange *(Citrus sinensis)*
3 drops Rosemary *(Rosmarinus officinalis ct. verbenone)*

Directions:
Mix oils together in small bowl and dip cotton wick into the mixture and let it absorb the oil blend. Place wick inside the blank inhaler and cap. Remove lid and place in nostril (closing off other nostril) and take several slow deep breaths. Repeat in other nostril. Use as often as needed energize.

Fatigue Fighter Aroma Inhaler

Materials:

blank inhaler
small glass mixing bowl

Ingredients:

6 drops Black Spruce *(Picea mariana)*
3 drops Atlas Cedarwood *(Cedrus atlantica)*
2 drops Peppermint *(Mentha X piperita)*

Directions:

Mix oils together in small bowl and dip cotton wick into the mixture and let it absorb the oil blend. Place wick inside the blank inhaler and cap. Remove lid and place in nostril (closing off other nostril) and take several slow deep breaths. Repeat in other nostril. Use as often as needed to fight fatigue.

Increase Your CHI Spritzer

Materials:

2 oz. dark glass bottle

Ingredients:

2 oz. peppermint hydrosol

6 drops Rosemary *(Rosmarinus officinalis ct. verbenone)*

5 drops Cypress *(Cupressus sempervirens)*

8 drops Cinnamon *(Cinnamomum zeylanicum)*

6 drops Eucalyptus *(Eucalyptus radiata)*

4 drops Thyme *(Thymus vulgaris ct linalol)*

10 drops Pink Grapefruit *(Citrus paradisi)*

Directions:

Combine all essential oils and mix thoroughly. Add to peppermint hydrosol and pour into 2 oz. glass bottle with spritzer top. Shake well. Spritz over head and shoulders avoiding eyes provide more vibrant energy.

Lively Foot Scrub

Materials:

small glass mixing bowl

Ingredients:

1/4 cup dead sea salt

1/3 cup extra virgin olive oil

10 drops Rosemary *(Rosmarinus officinalis ct. verbenone)*

6 drops Black Pepper *(Piper nigrum)*

2 drops Tea Tree *(Melaleuca alternifolia)*

Directions:

Mix all ingredients to form a loose paste. Apply to feet and rub in. Wrap feet in a warm wet towel and then in dry towel and let sit for 10 minutes. Rinse off with tepid water and pat dry. Feet will feel energized and refreshed.

Invigorating Shower Gel

Materials:

    4 oz. container with pump top
    small glass mixing bowl
    wire whisk

Ingredients:

    3.75 oz. unscented shower gel base (Nature's Sunshine - Sunshine Concentrate)
    2 tablespoons aloe vera gel
    2 teaspoons jojoba oil
    15 drops Pink Grapefruit *(Citrus paradisi)*
    10 drops Frankincense *(Boswelli carterii)*
    15 drops Eucalyptus *(Eucalyptus radiata)*
    10 drops Rosemary *(Rosmarinus officinalis ct. verbenone)*
    10 drops Peppermint *(Mentha x Piperita)*

Directions:

Whisk shower gel base, aloe vera gel and jojoba oil together. Add essential oils and mix thoroughly. Pour into 4 oz. container. Use several pumps on a shower scrunchie and lather up to invigorate and energize.

Take Control of Hot Flashes
& Night Sweats

The top essential oils for calming hot flashes are:

- Clary Sage

- Cypress

- Peppermint

- Geranium

Gone In A Flash Spritzer

Materials:

2 oz. dark glass bottle with spray top

Ingredients:

1.75 oz. peppermint hydrosol

.25 oz aloe vera gel

6 drops Peppermint *(Mentha X piperita)*

4 drops Geranium *(Pelargonium roseum x asperum)*

5 drops Clary Sage *(Salvia sclarea)*

3 drops Roman Chamomile *(Chamaemelum nobilis)*

8 drops Lemon *(Citrus limon)*

4 drops Cypress *(Cupressus sempervirens)*

Directions:

Mix the essential oils and aloe vera gel together and place in 2 oz. container. Add peppermint hydrosol, place the lid on and shake well. Spritz over face, neck and chest at the onset of a hot flash. Avoid eyes.

Menopause Relief Roll-On

This blend has saved me on more than one occasion. I used it for that agitated depression that can be difficult in the transition to menopause.

Materials:

1/3 oz. roll-on bottle

Ingredients:

1/3 oz. sweet almond oil

3 drops Geranium *(Pelargonium roseum x asperum)*

2 drops Lavender *(Lavandula angustifolia)*

3 drops Clary Sage *(Salvia sclarea)*

2 drops Sandalwood *(Santalum album)*

3 drops Peppermint *(Mentha X piperita)*

Directions:

Place the oils in the roll-on bottle and fill the remainder with sweet almond oil. Place the cap on and shake well to mix. Use on wrists, neck and temples for dealing with menopause symptoms.

Menopause Matters Massage Oil

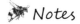

Materials:

    2 oz. dark glass bottle with treatment pump lid

Ingredients:

    1 oz. fractionated coconut oil

    1/2 oz. borage oil

    1/2 oz. evening primrose oil

    20 drops Rose Otto *(Rosa damascena)*

    7 drops Clary Sage *(Salvia sclarea)*

    3 drops Benzoin *(Styrax benzoin)*

Directions:

Blend all ingredients in a 2 oz. glass bottle. Place pumper lid on and shake well to mix. Use this oil to massage daily over abdomen or as a full body massage.

Cooling Spray

Aids in reducing hot flashes. I keep this one on my bedside table.

Materials:
    2 oz. glass bottle with spray top

Ingredients:
    2 oz. rose hydrosol
    8 drops Geranium *(Pelargonium roseum x asperum)*
    5 drops Pink Grapefruit *(Citrus paradisi)*
    5 drops Lime *(Citrus hystrix)*
    8 drops Palmarosa *(Cymbopogon martinii)*
    4 drop Peppermint *(Mentha X piperita)*

Directions:
Add essential oils in a 2 oz spray bottle of Rose hydrosol. Shake well before each use. Spritz above head (with eyes closed) when you feel a hot flash coming on.

"I couldn't be without the cooling spray. It stops my hot flashes in their tracks!"

               ~Lynn

Heart Palpitation Relief Roll-On

Heart palpitations are common during peri and menopause. This roll-on can support the heart and provide a sense of calm.

Materials:
    1/3 oz. roll-on bottle

Ingredients:
    1/3 oz. organic jojoba oil
    3 drops Neroli *(Citrus aurantium)*
    4 drops Rose Otto *(Citrus aurantium)*
    3 drops Ylang Ylang *(Cananga odorada)*

Directions:
Place the oils in the roll-on bottle and fill the remainder with jojoba oil. Place the cap on and shake well to mix. Use on wrists, neck and over the heart space.

Heart Soother

I have had personal success with this blend to relieve occasional heart palpitations associated with hot flashes and hormone imbalances.

Materials:

small glass mixing bowl

Ingredients:

1 tablespoon evening primrose oil
2 drops Neroli *(Citrus aurantium)*
1 drop Rose Otto *(Rosa damascena)*
2 drops Ylang Ylang *(Cananga Odorata)*

Directions:

Mix all ingredients together and massage over wrists, neck and heart space. Eliminating caffeine and alcohol from your diet will help as well.

PMS Relief

The top essential oils for PMS relief are:

- Geranium
- Clary Sage
- Thyme
- Ylang Ylang

Female Tonifying Massage Oil

Evening primrose is the superstar carrier oil in this blend. It provides the right synergy that invites the essential oils to sing in harmony.

Materials:

  2 oz. glass bottle with dropper top

Ingredients:

  1 1/2 oz. sweet almond oil
  1/2 oz. evening primrose oil
  2 vitamin E capsules
  10 drops Clary Sage *(Salvia sclarea)*
  8 drops Geranium *(Pelargonium roseum x asperum)*
  6 drops Lavender *(Lavandula angustifolia)*
  4 drops Palmarosa *(Cymbopogon martinii)*
  2 drops Sweet Marjoram *(Origanum marjorana)*

Directions:

Break open vitamin E capsules and mix all ingredients into a 2 oz. glass bottle. Place lid on and shake well. Massage into skin before bedtime daily. Relieves menstrual tension and cramping, headaches, insomnia, depression, irritability and mood swings.

PMS Roll-On

I've always kept one of these in my purse. I never travel without it.

Materials:
1/3 oz. roll-on bottle

Ingredients:
1/3 oz. sweet almond oil
5 drops Clary Sage *(Salvia sclarea)*
5 drops Lavender *(Lavandula angustifolia)*
2 drops Roman Chamomile *(Chamaemelum nobilis)*
3 drops Peppermint *(Mentha X piperita)*

Directions:
Place essential oils in 1/3 oz. roll-on ball bottle and fill remainder with sweet almond oil. Place cap on and shake well to mix. Roll over abdomen for menstrual cramping. Apply to temples and wrists to relieve headache, irritability & mood swings.

 Tip:

85% of American women experience PMS during peri-menopause

Women's Balance Lotion

This a great blend to support the female hormonal system and PMS.

Materials:
    2 oz. dark glass jar with lid

Ingredients:
    2 oz. organic unscented lotion
    7 drops Geranium *(Pelargonium roseum x asperum)*
    6 drops Lavender *(Lavandula angustifolia)*
    5 drops Cypress *(Cupressus sempervirens)*
    6 drops Clary Sage *(Salvia sclarea)*
    3 drops Rosemary *(Rosmarinus officinalis ct. verbenone)*
    3 drops Yarrow *(Achillea millefolium)*

Directions:
Combine the essential oils and unscented lotion in the jar. Stir well to combine. Massage a small amount of blend into abdomen area and lower back twice a day. Take a break from the using the blend during week of menstrual period if you still have a period.

Cramp Relief Oil

This cooling gel aids in reducing and eliminating menstrual cramping

Materials:
>2 oz. glass bottle with treatment pump top
>small glass mixing bowl

Ingredients:
>1.5 oz. aloe vera gel
>4 tsp. lobelia essence (Nature's Sunshine brand)
>6 drops Bergamot *(Citrus bergamia)*
>6 drops Roman Chamomile *(Chamaemelum nobilis)*
>5 drops Lavender *(Lavandula angustifolia)*
>4 drops Lemongrass *(Cymbopogon citratus)*
>4 drops Sweet Marjoram *(Origanum marjorana)*

Directions:
Mix aloe vera gel and lobelia essence together in a small mixing bowl and add essential oils. Mix well and place in glass bottle and put lid on. Apply gently to the area of cramping every 20 minutes until cramps subside.

Migraine Relief

Materials:

1 oz. dark glass bottle with treatment pump lid

Ingredients:

1 oz sweet almond oil

4 drops Peppermint *(Mentha X piperita)*

6 drops Tei fu (blend of Wintergreen, Menthol, Camphor, Clove, Eucalyptus, and Lavender essential oils) (Nature's Sunshine brand)

3 drops Roman Chamomile *(Chamaemelum nobilis)*

2 drops Helichrysum *(Helichrysum italicum)*

Directions:

Blend essential oils with sweet almond oil. Mix thoroughly, pour into container and place lid on. Shake well before each use. Rub over temples and back of neck every 10 minutes for relief.

PMS Rub

Materials:

1 oz. dark glass bottle with treatment pump lid

Ingredients:

1 oz sweet almond oil

2 drops Lavender *(Lavandula angustifolia)*

2 drops Roman Chamomile *(Chamaemelum nobilis)*

3 drops Geranium *(Pelargonium roseum x asperum)*

4 drops Clary Sage *(Salvia sclarea)*

3 drops Sandalwood *(Santalum album)*

2 drops Peppermint *(Mentha X piperita)*

Directions:

Blend essential oils with sweet almond oil. Mix thoroughly, pour into container and place lid on. Shake well before each use. Rub over abdomen and shoulders every 20 minutes to relieve PMS.

"I thought for sure I was going crazy when I entered menopause. Essential oils helped me get my emotions back on track. Thank you Angela."

~ Abby

PMS Mood Adjuster

Materials:

    2 oz. dark glass bottle with spray top

Ingredients:

    2 oz. rose hydrosol
    4 drops Neroli *(Citrus aurantium)*
    10 drops Pink Grapefruit *(Citrus paradisi)*
    8 drop Rose Otto *(Rosa damascena)*
    8 drops Sandalwood *(Santalum album)*

Directions:

Place all ingredients dark glass bottle and place cap on. Shake well to mix. Spritz over face and neck with eyes closed as needed to enhance mood, calm tension and relieve PMS.

Take The Edge Off

To relieve tension, pain and agitation

Materials:

    1/3 oz. roll-on container

Ingredients:

    1/3 oz. jojoba oil
    5 drops Frankincense *(Boswelli carterii)*
    2 drops Lemongrass *(Cymbopogon citratus)*
    3 drops Peppermint *(Mentha X piperita)*
    4 drops Rosewood *(Aniba roseodora)*

Directions:

Add essential oils to Jojoba oil and blend well. Place in roll-on bottle and put lid on. Apply to the back of your neck every 20 minutes to relieve headache tension and pain.

Headache Roll-On

Relieves headache tension, helps restore adrenals and reduces anxiety.

Materials:

 1/3 oz. roll-on bottle

Ingredients:

 1/3 oz. fractionated coconut oil
 2 drops Holy Basil *(Ocimum sanctum)*
 3 drops Lavender *(Lavandula angustifolia)*
 2 drops Peppermint *(Mentha X piperita)*
 3 drops Ylang ylang *(Cananga odorata)*

Directions:

Add essential oils to Jojoba oil and blend well. Place in roll-on bottle and put lid on. Gently massage in small circles over both temples, neck and shoulders every 20 minutes for the to relieve headache tension and pain.

Get a Good Night's Sleep

Sleep is essential for menopause health. Lack of sleep slowly erodes your immune system and can lead to increased cortisol and insulin levels. Make sleep a priority.

The top essential oils for improving sleep are:

- Lavender
- Sweet Marjoram
- Neroli

Sleep Ease Aroma Inhaler

Use throughout the evening to achieve the restful sleep you need at bedtime.

Materials:
blank inhaler
small glass mixing bowl

Ingredients:
2 drops Sweet Marjoram (*Origanum marjorana*)
2 drops Neroli (*Citrus aurantium*)
3 drops Lavender (*Lavandula angustifolia*)
4 drops Linden blossom (*Tilia vulgaris*)

Directions:
Mix oils together in small bowl and dip cotton wick into the mixture and let it absorb the oil blend. Place wick inside the blank inhaler and cap. Remove lid and place in nostril (closing off other nostril) and take several slow deep breaths. Repeat in other nostril. Use inhaler several times per hour throughout the evening before bedtime.

Kick Insomnia To The Curb

Materials:

2 oz. dark glass bottle with spray top

Ingredients:

1.75 oz organic witch hazel

4 droppers distress remedy homeopathic

8 drops Lavender *(Lavandula angustifolia)*

4 drops Sweet Marjoram *(Origanum marjorana)*

4 drops Roman Chamomile *(Chamaemelum nobilis)*

4 drops Patchouli *(Pogostemon cablin)*

3 drops Myrrh *(Commiphora myrrha)*

Directions:

Mix all ingredients together and place in 2 oz. dark glass bottle and place top on. Shake well before each use. Spritz over head and neck before bedtime, avoiding eyes and breathe deep. Keep by bedside and spritz if you wake up during the night.

Midnight Magic Spritzer

Materials:

2 oz. dark glass bottle with spray top

Ingredients:

10 drops Sweet Marjoram *(Origanum marjorana)*

14 drops Lavender *(Lavandula angustifolia)*

6 drops Roman Chamomile *(Chamaemelum nobilis)*

2 oz. witch hazel

Directions:

Mix all ingredients together and place in 2 oz. dark glass bottle and place top on. Shake well before each use. Spritz over head and neck before bedtime, avoiding eyes and breathe deep.

Nighty Night Sleep Tight - Diffuser Blend

Materials:

5ml amber bottle

Ingredients:

15 drops Lavender *(Lavandula angustifolia)*

10 drops Clary Sage *(Salvia sclarea)*

15 drops Ylang Ylang *(Cananga odorata)*

20 drops German Chamomile *(Matricaria recitita)*

20 drops Red Mandarin *(Citrus reticulata)*

20 drops Sandalwood *(Santalum album)*

Directions:

Mix all ingredients and place in 5ml amber bottle. Use several drops in a diffuser at night for restful sleep.

Restful Sleep Oil

Materials:
2 oz. dark glass bottle with dropper top

Ingredients:
2 oz. sweet almond oil
8 drops Bergamot *(Citrus bergamia)*
6 drops Red Mandarin *(Citrus reticulata)*
5 drops Ylang Ylang *(Cananga odorata)*
4 drops German Chamomile *(Matricaria recitita)*
4 drops Sweet Marjoram *(Origanum marjorana)*
3 drops Vetiver *(Vetiveria zizanoides)*

Directions:
Mix all ingredients together and place in the bottle with cap on and shake well. Place a few drops of oil in the palm of your hand and rub together briskly. Cup your hands over your nose and mouth and breathe deeply for several minutes. You can also rub the oil over your chest, shoulders and the bottoms of your feet before bed.

Sleep Lotion

Supports a deeper, calmer night's sleep

Materials:

    2 oz glass jar with lid

Ingredients:

    2 oz. organic unscented lotion
    4 drops Roman Chamomile *(Chamaemelum nobilis)*
    6 drops Rosewood *(Aniba roseodora)*
    4 drops Hyssop *(Hyssopus officinalis var. decumbens)*
    6 drops Melissa *(Melissa officinalis)*
    10 drops Linden Blossom *(Tilia vulgaris)*

Directions:

Add essential oils to 2 oz. of unscented lotion and mix well.
Apply to your chest, neck and bottoms of feet before bed.

Sleep Easy Gel

This gel not only helps improve sleep but it helps balance blood sugar and is cooling as well.

Materials:
> 2 oz. dark glass bottle with treatment pump
> small glass mixing bowl

Ingredients:
> .5 oz witch hazel
> 1.5 oz organic aloe vera gel
> 8 drops Sweet Orange *(Citrus sinensis)*
> 6 drops Lavender *(Lavandula angustifolia)*
> 6 drops Cinnamon *(Cinnamomum zeylanicum)*
> 4 drops Ylang ylang *(Cananga odorata)*
> 6 drops Atlas Cedarwood *(Cedrus atlantica)*

Directions:
Mix all ingredients together and put in glass bottle and place lid on. Shake well before each use. Use 2 pumps and gently massage in small circles over both temples, neck, shoulders and bottoms of feet before bed.

Enhance Libido and Improve Intimacy

The top essential oils for improving libido are:

- Jasmine

- Sandalwood

- Ylang Ylang

"In The Mood" Perfume Roll-On

Use throughout the evening to achieve the restful sleep you need at bedtime.

Materials:

1/3 roll-on bottle

Ingredients:

1/3 organic jojoba oil

3 drops Jasmine (*Jasminum grandiflorum*)

5 drops Sandalwood (*Santalum album*)

2 drops Ylang Ylang (*Cananga odorata*)

Directions:

Place 1/2 of the jojoba oil in the roll-on bottle then add the essential oils and fill roll-on bottle with the remaining jojoba oil. Place the work roller ball and lid on and shake well to mix all ingredients together. Use on wrists, neck and chest to invoke sensuality. You can also use this recipe to create a sensual massage blend.

Sensual Massage Blend 1

The aphrodisiac effect of this blend is perfect for a mutual massage to share with your partner

Materials:
  small glass mixing bowl

Ingredients:
  1 tablespoon grapeseed oil
  2 drops Ylang Ylang *(Cananga odorata)*
  3 drops Geranium *(Pelargonium roseum x asperum)*
  3 drops Sandalwood *(Santalum album)*

Directions:
Combine all ingredients and use for a full body massage.

Sensual Massage Blend 2

The aphrodisiac effect of this blend is perfect for a mutual massage to share with your partner

Materials:
  small glass mixing bowl

Ingredients:
  1 tablespoon fractionated coconut oil
  2 drops Jasmine *(Jasminum grandiflorum)*
  3 drops Rose Otto *(Rosa damascena)*
  3 drops Sandalwood *(Santalum album)*

Directions:
Combine all ingredients and use for a full body massage.

Perfect Lubrication Combination

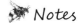

As peri-menopause approaches one of the first things we begin to notice is that we aren't a moist and juicy as we once were. This poses difficulties when it comes to intimacy. I discovered that organic hazelnut oil has the same pH as vaginal tissue which makes it an excellent lubricant. Caution: Do not use if you have nut allergies.

Materials:

    2 oz glass bottle with treatment pump lid

Ingredients:

    2 oz. organic hazelnut oil

    4 drops Lavender *(Lavandula angustifolia)*

    1 drop Neroli *(Citrus aurantium)*

    2 drop Rose Otto *(Rosa damascena)*

Directions:

Mix all ingredients together and place in bottle with lid on. Use several pumps as a lubricant before intimacy. This blend can also be used as a massage oil for intimacy.

Conquer Weight Management

Aromatherapy is the perfect companion to a weight loss program. Along with eating healthy foods and exercising, essential oils can play a vital role in balancing hormones and getting metabolism regulated.

The top essential oils for managing a healthy weight are:

- Pink Grapefruit

- Sweet Orange

- Cinnamon

- Fennel

 Tip:

Inhaling Pink Grapefruit oil 15 minutes before a meal curbs your appetite and let's you feel full so you won't overeat.

Appetite Suppressant

Use throughout the evening to achieve the restful sleep you need at bedtime.

Materials:
> 1 oz. dark glass bottle with dropper top

Ingredients:
> 1 oz sweet almond oil
> 8 drops distress remedy homeopathic
> 5 drops Bergamot *(Citrus bergamia)*
> 4 drops Coriander Seed *(Coriandrum sativum)*
> 6 drops Pink Grapefruit *(Citrus paradisi)*
> 1 drops Fennel, Sweet *(Foeniculum vulgare var. dulce)*

Directions:
Mix all ingredients in 1 oz. dark glass bottle and place dropper top on and shake well before each use. Apply a few drops to wrist, neck, throat and upper lip as needed to control appetite, food cravings and blood sugar.

Craving Calmer Aroma Inhaler

Keep this inhaler in your purse for those moments when will power is not enough

Materials:

blank inhaler
small glass mixing bowl

Ingredients:

6 drops Bergamot (*Citrus bergamia*)
6 drops Pink Grapefruit (*Citrus paradisi*)
3 drops Cinnamon (*Cinnamomum zeylanicum*)

Directions:

Mix essential oils together in a small glass container. Dip the cotton wick into the oils and let them all absorb into the wick. Place the wick in the blank inhaler and put the cap on. Twist cap off and place inhaler in one nostril as you close off the other nostril and repeat on the other side. Take several deep breaths on each side as needed when food cravings arise.

"When I incorporated essential oils into Angela's hormone balancing weight loss program it was a game changer for me. My mood improved and cravings vanished. I lost 15 pounds and feel fantastic!"

~ Janet

Crave FREE Roll-On

Just the perfect solution for reducing those cravings for sugar and carbs with the added benefit of hormone balancing.

Materials:

    1/3 oz. roll-on bottle

Ingredients:

    1/3 oz. organic jojoba oil

    15 drops Geranium *(Pelargonium roseum x asperum)*

Directions:

Place all ingredients in roll-on bottle, place roller ball and lid on and shake well. Apply to the bottoms of your feet morning and night and be Crave FREE from sugar and carbs.

Insulin Balancing Diffuser Blend

Materials:

    5 ml dark glass bottle

Ingredients:

    40 drops Cinnamon leaf *(Cinnamomum zeylanicum)*

    20 drops Geranium *(Pelargonium roseum x asperum)*

    8 drops Ylang Ylang *(Cananga odorata)*

    12 drops Eucalyptus *(Eucalyptus radiata)*

    20 drops Bergamot *(Citrus bergamia)*

Directions:

Mix essential oils together and place in 5ml dark glass bottle with lid on. Put several drops of the blend in a diffuser throughout the day to aid in balancing blood sugars and fighting insulin resistance. You can also take 2 drops of this blend in 1 teaspoon of carrier oil and rub over pancreas area (left side just below the ribcage) three times a day.

Appetite Control Aroma Inhaler

This inhaler aids in appetite control and reduces anxiety around dieting and food restriction. It stimulates the body to feel full and satisfied between meals while supporting healthy digestion. This blend also has essential oils in it to keep you grounded and focused on your goal and intention to lose weight. You won't want to be without this blend for successful weight loss!

Materials:

    blank inhaler

    small glass mixing bowl

Ingredients:

    3 drops Bergamot *(Citrus bergamia)*

    2 drops Neroli *(Citrus aurantium)*

    3 drops Pink Grapefruit *(Citrus paradisi)*

    1 drop Patchouli *(Pogostemon cablin)*

    1 drop Fennel *(Foeniculum vulgare var. dulce)*

    1 drop Vetiver *(Vetiveria zizanoides)*

Directions:

Mix essential oils in small glass bowl and place cotton wick in bowl to absorb oils. Place wick in blank inhaler and place cap on. To use remove cap and place in one nostril while closing the other nostril. Take several deep slow breaths and switch to the other nostril. Use the Appetite Control Inhaler 10 minutes before each meal to allow the body to feel more satiated and to support digestive health.

Weight Away Diffuser Blend

This blend is not only refreshing and uplifting but has ingredients with research behind it for weight loss. The key ingredient is pink grapefruit essential oil. In research studies Pink Grapefruit oil helps initiate the hormone leptin or satiation hormone. This make you feel full sooner and satisfied with eating less.

Materials:

5ml dark glass bottle

Ingredients:

40 drops Pink Grapefruit *(Citrus paradisi)*

35 drops Sweet Orange *(Citrus sinensis)*

25 drops Lemon *(Citrus limon)*

3 drops Fennel *(Foeniculum vulgare var. dulce)*

Directions:

Mix essential oils together and place in 5ml bottle. Use 3-4 drops in a diffuser throughout the day to balance leptin and reduce urges to snack.

Weight Away Aroma Inhaler

This inhaler is like your "power" stick. Take it anywhere and everywhere to help you stay focused on your weight loss goals, feel more satisfied with less food and have your mood and blood sugar balanced. Perfect for the occasional detox headaches that you might experience while trying to lose weight or get off of caffeine.

Materials:

blank inhaler
small glass mixing bowl

Ingredients:

7 drops Pink Grapefruit *(Citrus paradisi)*
4 drops Peppermint *(Mentha X piperita)*

Directions:

Mix oils together in small bowl and dip cotton wick into the mixture and let it absorb the oil blend. Place wick inside the blank inhaler and cap. Remove lid and place in nostril (closing off other nostril) and take several slow deep breaths. Repeat in other nostril.

Hair & Skincare Essentials

Moving into peri-menopause and menopause you start to notice changes to your skin and hair. Here are some great ways to keep your hair and skin glowing.

The top essential oils for hair and skincare are:

- Neroli
- Atlas Cedarwood
- Rosemary
- Lavender

Love The Skin You're In - Body Lotion

This silky smooth lotion nourishes the skin while balancing hormones

Materials:
2 oz. dark glass container

Ingredients:
2 oz. organic unscented lotion
10 drops Bergamot *(Citrus bergamia)*
6 drops Clary Sage *(Salvia sclarea)*
6 drops Geranium *(Pelargonium roseum x asperum)*
8 drops Palmarosa *(Cymbopogon martinii)*

Directions:
Mix essential oils into lotion base and store in glass jar. Apply morning and night to abdomen and inner thighs to assist in balancing hormones.

Caution:
Citrus oils are photosensitive so use caution with sun exposure after use.

"Since I have been receiving hand reflexology using Angela's expertise and special blends of essential oils, I have noticed a remarkable difference in my skin and my mood for the remainder of the week. She chooses oils based upon what I am feeling both physiologically and psychologically in order for my experience to be most effective. Her skills and the continual use of her products have not only alleviated the eczema on my hands, but have also reduced my stress levels immediately after our sessions."

~Sam

Rosacea Remedy

Materials:
>   2 oz. dark glass bottle with spray top

Ingredients:
>   2 oz. rose hydrosol
>   4 drops Rose Otto *(Rosa damascena)*
>   6 drops Lavender *(Lavandula angustifolia)*

Directions:

Mix all ingredients in glass bottle and place lid on. Shake well and spritz areas where rosacea appears (usually on cheeks and nose) two times a day.

 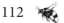

Cellulite Buster

Best results when used after dry brushing skin and showering

Materials:

1 oz. glass bottle with treatment pump lid

Ingredients:

1/2 oz. pomegranate seed oil

1/2 oz. sweet almond oil

6 drops Pink Grapefruit *(Citrus paradisi)*

3 drops Geranium *(Pelargonium roseum x asperum)*

3 drops Lemon *(Citrus limon)*

1 drops Thyme *(Thymus vulgaris ct linalol)*

2 drop Oregano *(Origanum vulgare)*

Directions:

Mix all ingredients together and place in glass bottle with treatment pump lid. Apply a few pumps in the palm of your hand. Rub hands together briskly to warm. Massage into areas of cellulite daily after showering.

Edema Ease

Hormonal changes can cause edema. I love the essential oil Cypress and Lemongrass to help ease edema because they move stagnation and help eliminate excess fluids.

Materials:

small glass mixing bowl

Ingredients:

1 cup epsom salts or magnesium flakes

1 teaspoon sweet almond oil

4 drops Cypress *(Cupressus sempervirens)*

2 drops Lemongrass *(Cymbopogon citratus)*

6 drops Lavender *(Lavandula angustifolia)*

2 drops Atlas Cedarwood *(Cedrus atlantica)*

1 drop Frankincense *(Boswelli carterii)*

Directions:

Add salts to small bowl and mix in essential oils and sweet almond oil. Add to warm bath and soak for 15-20 minutes. After the bath, create a massage blend with 1 tablespoon sweet almond oil and 3 drops helichrysum *(Helichrysum italicum)*. Massage over area of edema. For a more stimulating effect, add 1 drop Cinnamon Leaf *(Cinnamomum zeylanicum)* or 1 drop Rosemary *(Rosmarinus officinalis ct. verbenone)* to the massage blend.

No More Pain And Inflammation Creme

Reduces muscular pain and inflammation

Materials:
　　2 oz. dark glass jar
　　double boiler

Ingredients:
　　1/2 oz. shea butter
　　1/2 oz. jojoba oil
　　1/2 oz. arnica infused oil
　　1/4 oz. beeswax pastilles
　　8 drops Balsam Copiaba (*Copaiba balsamifera*)
　　5 drops German Chamomile (*Matricaria recitita*)
　　5 drops Helichrysum (*Helichrysum italicum*)
　　8 drops Lavender (*Lavandula angustifolia*)
　　4 drops Lemongrass (*Cymbopogon citratus*)

Directions:
Melt shea butter, jojoba oil and arnica oil and beeswax in a double boiler. Remove from heat and allow to cool slightly. Add essential oils and stir. Pour into glass jar and allow to cool before placing lid on. Rub salve on achy muscles to relieve pain and inflammation.

Anti-Inflammatory Oil

Alleviates inflammation and pain

Materials:

> 2 oz. dark glass bottle with treatment pump lid
> small glass mixing bowl

Ingredients:

> 1 oz. tamanu oil
> 1 oz. baobab oil
> 6 drops German Chamomile *(Matricaria recitita)*
> 10 drops Frankincense *(Boswelli carterii)*
> 6 drops Helichrysum *(Helichrysum italicum)*
> 6 drops Lavender *(Lavandula angustifolia)*
> 4 drops Sandalwood *(Santalum album)*
> 4 drops Rosemary *(Rosmarinus officinalis ct. verbenone)*

Directions:

Blend essential oils with tamanu and baobab oils. Mix thoroughly, pour into container and place lid on. Shake well before each use. Gently apply to inflamed area 3-4 times daily. Caution: Do not use on open wounds.

Scalp Treatment For Hair Loss

Materials:

Warming pot

Ingredients:

1 tablespoon organic jojoba oil

2 teaspoons sweet almond oil

8 drops Lavender *(Lavandula angustifolia)*

5 drops Clary Sage *(Salvia sclarea)*

3 drops Rosemary *(Rosmarinus officinalis ct. verbenone)*

3 drops Ylang Ylang *(Cananga odorata)*

Directions:

Place ingredients in the warming pot. Stir well and warm up. Put on hair and work into the scalp. Wrap hair in a dry towel and let set overnight 3-4 times a week. Shampoo out with warm water in the morning and style as usual.

"I love the skin care products Angela has created! They are lightly scented and make my face feel wonderful. I only wish I knew about them years ago! Thank you Angela."

~ Dianne

No More Wrinkles

Materials:

 2 oz. glass bottle with treatment pump lid

Ingredients:

 1 oz. apricot kernel oil

 .5 oz. pomegranate seed oil

 .5 oz. rosehip seed oil

 1 vitamin E capsule

 10 drops Geranium *(Pelargonium roseum x asperum)*

 6 drops Frankincense *(Boswelli carterii)*

 8 drops Carrot Seed *(Daucus carota)*

 4 drops Ylang Ylang *(Cananga odorata)*

Directions:

Mix all ingredients together and place in glass bottle with lid on. After washing your face, use 2 pumps in the palm of your hand. Rub briskly to warm the oil and apply to face using circular upwards motions until absorbed.

Abundant Hair Formula

Materials:

2 oz. dark glass bottle with dropper bottle lid

Ingredients:

1.5 oz. fractionated coconut oil

.5 oz. organic extra virgin olive oil

1 teaspoon hexane free castor oil

8 drops Peppermint *(Mentha X piperita)*

4 drops Rosemary *(Rosmarinus officinalis ct. verbenone)*

6 drops Geranium *(Pelargonium roseum x asperum)*

6 drops Lavender *(Lavandula angustifolia)*

2 drops Pine Needle *(Pinus sylvestris)*

3 drops Clary Sage *(Salvia sclarea)*

Directions:

Mix all ingredients together in dark glass bottle. Use 1 dropper full daily and rub into scalp to stimulate new hair growth.

 Tip:

In a recent study, peppermint essential oil was shown to regrow hair better than the prescription drug Rogaine.

Luscious Locks Hair Tonic

Encourages new hair growth

Materials:

quart glass jar
Squeeze bottle with a pointed lid

Ingredients:

4 cups boiling water
2 tablespoons fenugreek seeds
6 drops Clary Sage *(Salvia sclarea)*
6 drops Peppermint *(Mentha X piperita)*
6 drops Rosemary *(Rosmarinus officinalis ct. verbenone)*

Directions:

Place fenugreek seeds in quart jar. Heat water to boiling and pour over the seeds. Let steep overnight. Strain out the seeds and add the essential oils. FIll squeeze bottle and keep in the shower. Store the remaining mixture in the refrigerator. After washing your hair squeeze mixture on your scalp and let sit for a few minutes. Rinse out with cool water.

Liver Detoxification & Digestion

The top essential oils for detoxing the liver and digestive issues are:

- Pink Grapefruit
- Lemon
- Rosemary
- Ginger
- Thyme
- Palmarosa
- Roman Chamomile
- Lavender

Liver Tonic Roll-On

Supports both liver and bile duct

Materials:
    1/3 oz. roll-on bottle

Ingredients:
    1/3 oz. organic jojoba oil
    6 drops Geranium *(Pelargonium roseum x asperum)*
    4 drops Clary Sage *(Salvia sclarea)*
    4 drops Green Myrtle *(Myrtus communis)*

Directions:
Place all ingredients in roll-on bottle and place roller ball and lid on and shake well to mix. Roll over liver area (right side under rib cage) several times a day.

"I've had difficulties with my liver since I was in my 40's. With the essential oil roll-ons I have seen a big improvement in being able to digest fats."

~ Barbara

Liver Detox Roll-On

Materials:

    1/3 oz. roll-on bottle

Ingredients:

    1/3 oz. hexane free castor oil

    2 drops German Chamomile *(Matricaria recitita)*

    3 drops Carrot Seed *(Daucus carota)*

    4 drops Helichrysum *(Helichrysum italicum)*

    10 drops Bitter Orange *(Citrus aurantium)*

Directions:

Mix all ingredients in 1/3 oz. roll-on bottle and place roller ball and lid on and shake well to mix. Roll over liver area (right side under rib cage) several times a day.

Castor Oil Pack

When I'm feeling sluggish I do a castor oil pack a few nights a week before bed and it's incredibly rejuvenating and beneficial for peri-menopause and menopause.

- Improves Digestion, Assimilation and Relieves Constipation

- Aids in Hormonal Balance (PMS for Women)

- Detoxifies your Organs, Tissues, and Joints

- Helps Reduce Inflammation and Pain

- Supports and Reduces Stiffness and Arthritis

- Stimulates the Liver, Lymphatic System, and the Immune System

Materials:
    small glass mixing bowl
    wool flannel sheet
    hot water bottle or heating pad

Ingredients:
    1 oz. hexane free castor oil
    3 drops Lemon *(Citrus limon)*
    4 drops Pink Grapefruit *(Citrus paradisi)*
    2 drops Ginger *(Zingiber officinale)*
    2 drops Thyme *(Thymus vulgaris ct linalol)*
    2 drops Oregano *(Origanum vulgare)*
    2 drops Rosemary *(Rosmarinus officinalis ct. verbenone)*

Directions:
Mix all ingredients in small glass bowl and mix thoroughly. Place the mixture onto the wool flannel sheet. Place the sheet on your liver, which is located directly under your right rib-

cage. Lay down in bed with a towel under you so that the oily flannel doesn't accidentally get on the sheets. Then, place another towel over the castor oil pack before placing the hot water bottle or heating pad on top. Use an old towel that you don't mind getting stained. Leave it on for 15-20 minutes.

Caution: DO NOT do castor oils packs during your period if you are still menstruating. Do them before or after your period.

Detoxifying Bath

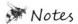

This detox bath is very effective for removing toxins and soaking away aches and pains.

Materials:

2 small glass mixing bowls

Ingredients:

1/2 cup bentonite clay

1/2 cup epsom salts, magnesium flakes or sea salts

1 teaspoon sweet almond oil

3 drops Lemon *(Citrus limon)*

3 drops Bergamot *(Citrus bergamia)*

3 drops Pink Grapefruit *(Citrus paradisi)*

3 drops Thyme *(Thymus vulgaris ct linalol)*

Directions:

Before you take a bath, dry brush your skin and rinse. Mix essential oils and sweet almond oil in a glass mixing bowl. Mix salt and clay in a separate glass bowl. Pour essential oil mixture into the salt and clay mixture and add to bath water. Soak 15-20 minutes. Rinse off. Baths are very effective for removing toxins and soaking away aches and pains.

"The way to health is to have an aromatic bath and a scented massage every day."

~ Hippocrates

Relaxing Detox Bath

Materials:

small glass mixing bowl

Ingredients:

1 cup epsom salts or magnesium flakes

1 teaspoon sweet almond oil

6 drops Lemon *(Citrus limon)*

1 drop Thyme *(Thymus vulgaris ct linalol)*

2 drop Rose Otto *(Rosa damascena)*

Directions:

Place salt in bowl and add essential oils and sweet almond oil.
Mix well and add to warm bath and soak 15-20 minutes.

Digest Well

Eases digestion and may assist in preventing gas & bloating

Materials:

2 oz. jar with lid

Ingredients:

2 oz. organic unscented lotion

1 drop Bergamot *(Citrus bergamia)*

3 drops Cardamom *(Elettaria cardamomum)*

3 drops Roman Chamomile *(Chamaemelum nobilis)*

2 drops Sweet Orange *(Citrus sinensis)*

Directions:

Blend essential oils in 2 oz of unscented lotion. Rub over your
stomach area before every meal and before bed.

Cramps Be Gone

This blend works well for intestinal cramping and bloating

Materials:

1 oz. glass bottle with dropper top

Ingredients:

1 oz. sweet almond oil

4 drops Bergamot *(Citrus bergamia)*

5 drops Peppermint *(Mentha X piperita)*

2 drops Clove *(Eugenia caryophyllata)*

4 drops Roman Chamomile *(Chamaemelum nobilis)*

Directions:

Mix all ingredients in glass bottle. Place dropper top on and shake well. Use one dropper full and rub on abdomen to relieve cramping.

IBS Relief Roll-On

I found this blend so helpful when I was in peri-menopause and my digestive system was a wreck.

Materials:
1/3 oz. roll-on bottle

Ingredients:
1/3 oz. sweet almond oil

3 drops Bergamot *(Citrus bergamia)*

2 drops Roman Chamomile *(Chamaemelum nobilis)*

2 drops Peppermint *(Mentha X piperita)*

2 drops Clary Sage *(Salvia sclarea)*

2 drops Thyme *(Thymus vulgaris ct linalol)*

Directions:
Place all ingredients in roll-on bottle and place roller ball and lid on. Shake well to blend. Rub over abdomen as needed to soothe bloating, cramping and IBS symptoms.

Adrenal Support

The top essential oils for supporting the adrenals are:

- Holy Basil
- Geranium
- Nutmeg
- Black Spruce

Adrenal Support Roll-On

Nutmeg essential oil increases melatonin and supports the adrenals

Materials:

1/3 oz. roll-on bottle

Ingredients:

1/3 oz. grapeseed oil
15 drops Nutmeg (*Myristica fragrans*)

Directions:

Place all ingredients in roll-on bottle and place roller ball and lid on and shake well. Roll over adrenal glands (low back above the kidneys) AM & PM for support.

Bedtime Adrenal Support Lotion

This adrenal restorative lotion helps manage stress, enhances sleep and reduces anxiety.

Materials:

2 oz. glass jar with lid

small glass mixing bowl

whisk

Ingredients:

2 oz. unscented organic lotion base

12 drops Linden blossom *(Tilia vulgaris)*

6 drops of Lavender *(Lavandula angustifolia)*

6 drops of Atlas Cedarwood *(Cedrus atlantica)*

6 drops of Rose Otto *(Rosa damascena)*

Directions:

Add the essential oils to the lotion in the mixing bowl and whisk well. Place lotion in jar and place lid on tightly. Rub over your adrenal glands, using gentle, circular motions several times a day. The adrenal glands are located just above your kidneys, on your lower back.

Adrenal Support Spritzer

Combats fatigue and that mid afternoon energy slump

Materials:

   2 oz. dark glass bottle with spray topper

Ingredients:

   2 oz tulsi holy basil hydrosol
   10 drops silver shield (colloidal silver)
   8 drops German Chamomile *(Matricaria recitita)*
   6 drops Green Mandarin *(Citrus reticulata var. mandarine)*
   6 drops Benzoin *(Styrax benzoin)*

Directions:

Combine all ingredients in 2 oz. glass bottle and place spray top on and shake well. Spritz above your head, closing your eyes and taking deep breaths several times per day to support adrenals and combat exhaustion and fatigue. For additional support, spritz over low back and rub in.

Adrenal Support Massage Oil

Materials:
  2 oz. dark glass bottle with treatment pump top

Ingredients:
  2 oz. sweet almond oil
  5 drops Black Spruce *(Picea mariana)*
  5 drops Pine Needle *(Pinus sylvestris)*
  5 drops Cypress *(Cupressus sempervirens)*
  5 drops Sweet Orange *(Citrus sinensis)*

Directions:
Mix all ingredients together and place in dark glass bottle with lid on tightly. Use two pumps of the blend in the palm of your hand and rub   between hands to create some friction and warmth and then rub over adrenal/kidney area on low back three times a day for adrenal support.

"The reflexology points really made a difference for me. Before I started using essential oils on my feet they were always tender, now I could dance all night and have the energy to do it."

~ Marianne

Reflexology Adrenal Support Blend

This blend is very effective when used on the adrenal reflexes on the foot.

Materials:

1/3 oz. roll-on bottle

Ingredients:

1/3 oz. jojoba oil

6 drops Pine Needle *(Pinus sylvestris)*

4 drops Lavender *(Lavandula angustifolia)*

3 drop Roman Chamomile *(Chamaemelum nobilis)*

Directions:

Mix all ingredients in roll-on bottle, place roller ball and cap on and shake to blend well. Apply to arches of feet morning and evening.

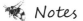

Genitourinary Support

The top essential oils for genitourinary support are:

- Lavender

- Rose Otto

- Geranium

Leaky Bladder

Materials:

    5 ml dark bottle

Ingredients:

    45 drops Lavender *(Lavandula angustifolia)*
    25 drops Bergamot *(Citrus bergamia)*
    30 drops Lemon *(Citrus limon)*

Directions:

Combine oils into 5ml bottle. Mix 5 to 10 drops of the blend with a cup of Epsom Salts. Place in the tub and soak at least 3 times a week. Massage the feet after each bath with three drops of the blend mixed in 1 teaspoon of carrier oil. Focus on the inner arch of the foot where the bladder reflexology point is located. Or diffuse 5-10 drops of the blend for 5 minutes before bed.

Bladder Rescue Rub

This blend helps relieve bladder infections and cystitis

Materials:
small glass mixing bowl

Ingredients:
1/2 oz. fractionated coconut oil
5 drops Bergamot (*Citrus bergamia*)
2 drops Sandalwood (*Santalum album*)
3 drops Tea Tree (*Melaleuca alternifolia*)
2 drops Thyme (*Thymus vulgaris ct linalol*)
1 drop Frankincense (*Boswelli carterii*)

Directions:
Mix all ingredients and massage into low back area and abdomen several times a day.

 Tip:

Fluctuating hormones can leave you vulnerable to bladder and yeast infections

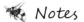

Diuretic Lotion

Aids in reduction of excess fluids

Materials:

2 oz. glass jar

small glass mixing bowl

Ingredients:

2 oz. unscented lotion

5 drops Cypress *(Cupressus sempervirens)*

4 drops Frankincense *(Boswelli carterii)*

5 drops Pink Grapefruit *(Citrus paradisi)*

5 drops Juniper Berry *(Juniperus communis)*

3 drops Bay Laurel *(Laurus nobilis)*

3 drops Lemon *(Citrus limon)*

Directions:

Blend essential oils into 2 oz of unscented lotion and pour in to glass jar. Apply gently to puffy areas such as ankles or hands 3-4 times daily.

Vaginal Health - how to heal and nourish the pelvic floor. I recommend that any woman who has had a child vaginally or had trauma that involves the pelvic floor such as a car accident or sexual violence to go see a physical therapist that specializes in pelvic floor work. I've had several sessions with an amazing practitioner in Portland, Oregon by the name of Tami Lynn Kent. She recently did a TEDx Portland talk called the Vagina Whisperer. You can watch it on YouTube. Her book is entitled *Wild Feminine*. Tami's work enabled me to eliminate vaginal dryness, have better sex and feel more comfortable in my feminine wisdom as I moved through menopause.

Vaginal Moisturizer/Lubricant

Materials:

Small glass container

Ingredients:

1 tablespoon organic hazelnut oil

2 tablespoons aloe vera gel

2 drops Jasmine *(Jasminum grandiflorum)* or Neroli *(Citrus aurantium)* or Ylang Ylang *(Cananga odorata)*

Directions:

Mix all ingredients together and apply to your delicate parts to moisturize or use as a lubricant.

Vulva/Perineum Soothing Pads

Materials:

Cosmetic pads

2 oz. glass jar

Ingredients:

.5 oz aloe vera gel

.5 oz organic witch hazel

.5 oz organic hazelnut oil

(if allergic to nuts use jojoba oil)

4 drops Rose Otto *(Rosa damascena)*

Directions:

Mix all ingredients well in small glass bowl. Add cosmetic pads to glass jar and pour mixture over the pads, making sure to saturate all pads. Place lid on and store in cool, dry place. Use daily or after sex to soothe the vulva and perineum.

Vaginosis Sitz Bath Blend

Aids in the relief of vaginal infections

Materials:
   small glass mixing bowl

Ingredients:
   1 cup epsom salts or magnesium flakes
   1 teaspoon sweet almond oil
   3 drops Geranium *(Pelargonium roseum x asperum)*
   2 drops Tea Tree *(Melaleuca alternifolia)*
   3 drops Lavender *(Lavandula angustifolia)*
   2 drops Roman Chamomile *(Chamaemelum nobilis)*

Directions:
Mix essential oils and sweet almond oil with epsom salts and soak your delicate parts in a shallow bath (3-6 inches of warm water) for 15-20 minutes for several days.

Vaginosis Salve

Materials:

1 oz. glass container

Ingredients:

1 oz. golden salve (Nature's Sunshine brand)

4 probiotic capsules (I recommend Jarro-Dophilus vaginal probiotics for women)

3 drops Geranium (*Pelargonium roseum x asperum*)

2 drops Tea Tree (*Melaleuca alternifolia*)

4 drops Lavender (*Lavandula angustifolia*)

2 drops Roman Chamomile (*Chamaemelum nobilis*)

4 drops Palmarosa (*Cymbopogon martinii*)

Directions:

Stir the essential oils into the golden salve container and open the probiotic capsules and add them to the mixture. Apply to vulva and vaginal area after a vaginosis sitz bath before bedtime.

Cautions and contraindications: Discontinue use if irritation occurs.

Vaginal Suppositories

Suppositories can be used for vaginal infections (vaginal candida), vaginal irritation and/or dryness. It also soothes herpes outbreaks.

Materials:

small glass mixing bowl
plastic wrap or aluminum foil
container with lid

Ingredients:

2 oz. golden salve (Nature's Sunshine brand)
6 probiotic capsules (I recommend Jarro-Dophilus vaginal probiotics for women)
12 drops Lavender *(Lavandula angustifolia)*
5 drops Myrrh *(Commiphora myrrha)*
4 drops Tea Tree *(Melaleuca alternifolia)*
5 drops Geranium *(Pelargonium roseum x asperum)*
4 drops Rose Otto *(Rosa damascena)*

Directions:

In a small mixing bowl, open the probiotic capsules and add all other ingredients. Mix well. Cover mixture and place in refrigerator for 1 hour or until mixture gets firm. Remove from refrigerator and scoop out 1 1/2 teaspoons at a time and form into small egg shaped suppositories. Individually wrap them loosely in foil or plastic wrap. Place in a container and store in the freezer for up to 3 months. Use as needed for vaginal infections, candida, irritation or dryness.

Candida

Dealing with Candida and yeast overgrowth takes persistence and patience. In addition to using essential oils here are some herbs & supplements to consider: caprylic acid, olive leaf extract, garlic, acidophilus, bifidophilus, pau d' arco, olive oil, vitamin C, B-Complex. In additions, eliminate all sugar from your diet including fruit.

Candida-Free Sitz Bath

This is a great way to help your body eliminate yeast overgrowth

Materials:
　small glass mixing bowl

Ingredients:
　1 teaspoon castile soap
　2 tablespoons apple cider vinegar
　2 drops Tea Tree *(Melaleuca alternifolia)*
　2 drops Sandalwood *(Santalum album)*
　1 drop Thyme *(Thymus vulgaris ct linalol)*
　2 drops Lavender *(Lavandula angustifolia)*

Directions:
Mix castile soap and essential oils together then add apple cider vinegar. Put mixture into 3-6 inches of warm bath water. Soak for 15-20 minutes for several days in a row to combat candida and yeast overgrowth.

 Tip:

A topical application will absorb up to 60% of the essential oil through the skin.

Candida Immune Boost Massage Oil

Materials:

 2 oz. glass bottle with dropper top

Ingredients:

 2 oz. grapeseed oil

 4 drops Lemon *(Citrus limon)*

 7 drops Tea Tree *(Melaleuca alternifolia)*

 5 drops Thyme *(Thymus vulgaris ct linalol)*

 3 drops Rosemary *(Rosmarinus officinalis ct. verbenone)*

 2 drops Geranium *(Pelargonium roseum x asperum)*

 2 drops Lavender *(Lavandula angustifolia)*

Directions:

Mix all ingredients in glass bottle. Place dropper top on and shake well. Use 1-2 droppers full as a daily massage oil for your lower abdomen and delicate feminine parts.

The Candida Solution

This protocol has worked for me personally.

Materials:

00 Gel Capsules

Ingredients:

2 teaspoons organic extra virgin olive oil

1 drop Oregano *(Origanum vulgare)*

1 drop Tea Tree *(Melaleuca alternifolia)*

1 drop Myrrh *(Commiphora myrrha)*

1 drop Cinnamon Bark *(Cinnamomum zeylanicum)*

1 drop Palmarosa *(Cymbopogon martinii)*

Directions:

Combine all ingredients. Using an eye dropper, fill the 00 gel capsules with the mixture and take twice daily for 10 days then stop for 10 days and repeat. I like to make up 10 days worth and keep them in the refrigerator in an airtight container so I don't need to make them up each day.

Fibroid Fighter

Materials:

1 oz. glass jar with lid

Ingredients:

1 oz. golden salve (Nature's Sunshine brand)

6 drops Lavender *(Lavandula angustifolia)*

3 drops Frankincense *(Boswelli carterii)*

2 drops Myrrh *(Commiphora myrrha)*

3 drops Geranium *(Pelargonium roseum x asperum)*

2 drops Rose Otto *(Rosa damascena)*

2 drops Sandalwood *(Santalum album)*

Directions:

Mix the essential oils into the golden salve and place in a 1 oz glass container. Rub over uterus or ovaries daily to help with cysts. For best results also look at stress levels and diet. Eliminate red meat, sugar, caffeine and alcohol from your diet.

Thyroid Support

The top essential oils for thyroid support are:

- Myrrh
- Lemongrass
- Thyme
- Clove

Thyroid Support Roll-On

Materials:

1/3 oz. roll-on bottle

Ingredients:

1/3 oz. jojoba oil
3 drops Frankincense *(Boswelli carterii)*
3 drops Myrrh *(Commiphora myrrha)*
2 drops Lemongrass *(Cymbopogon citratus)*
1 drop Clove *(Eugenia caryophyllata)*
1 drop Peppermint *(Mentha X piperita)*

Directions:

Mix all ingredients together and place in roll-on bottle. Apply to thyroid area on the front of the neck several times a day.

"I've used the thyroid roll-on for 3 months. At my last appointment the doctor said my nodules had reduced. I'm so pleased."

~ Allison

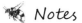

Reflexology Blend For Thyroid Support

Materials:

2 oz. glass bottle with treatment pump lid

Ingredients:

1 oz. tamanu oil

1 oz. grapeseed oil

8 drops Frankincense *(Boswelli carterii)*

7 drops Myrrh *(Commiphora myrrha)*

5 drops Lemongrass *(Cymbopogon citratus)*

5 drops Thyme *(Thymus vulgaris ct linalol)*

5 drops Holy Basil *(Ocimum sanctum)*

Directions:

Mix all ingredients and place in 2 oz. glass bottle with treatment pump lid. Apply several pumps each night to the soles of the feet before bedtime. Rub in the area between the ball of the foot and the big toe and all around the base of the big toe. This is where the reflexology points are for the thyroid.

Thyroid Maintenance Lotion

This lotion will help with low thyroid symptoms. It moves stagnation out, boosts energy and fights fatigue.

Materials:

2 oz. jar with lid

Ingredients:

2 oz. organic unscented lotion
Lemongrass (*Cymbopogon citratus*)
Spearmint (Mentha spicata)
Lemon (*Citrus limon*)
Frankincense (*Boswelli carterii*)
Rosemary (*Rosmarinus officinalis ct. verbenone*)

Directions:

Mix all ingredients together. Apply to neck, chest and arms daily.

Immune Enhancement

The top essential oils for immune system support are:

- Tea Tree
- Thyme
- Lemon
- Rosemary

 Tip:

Immune system health is one of the pillars of hormone balance

Immune Support Aroma Inhaler

Materials:
blank inhaler
small glass mixing bowl

Ingredients:
4 drops Eucalyptus *(Eucalyptus radiata)*
4 drops Tea Tree *(Melaleuca alternifolia)*
5 drops Black Spruce *(Picea mariana)*

Directions:
Mix oils together in small bowl and dip cotton wick into the mixture and let it absorb the oil blend. Place wick inside the blank inhaler and cap. Remove lid and place in nostril (closing off other nostril) and take several slow deep breaths. Repeat in other nostril. Use as often as needed for immune support.

Immune Support Lotion

Materials:

2 oz. jar with lid

Ingredients:

2 oz. organic unscented lotion

6 drops Lavender *(Lavandula angustifolia)*

10 drops Lemon *(Citrus limon)*

6 drops Palmarosa *(Cymbopogon martinii)*

6 drops Thyme *(Thymus vulgaris ct linalol)*

Directions:

Mix essential oils into lotion base and store in glass jar. Apply morning and night to throat and chest to strengthen the immune system and balance thyroid.

Tip:

In the fall get a jump start on cold and flu season by strengthening the immune system and detoxing the body. Begin with dry skin brushing (use a natural bristle brush) to encourage lymphatic movement and follow up with the lymphatic massage blend.

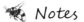

Lymphatic Massage Blend

This blend aids in supporting lymphatic movement and strengthening the immune system.

Materials:

    2 oz. glass bottle with treatment pump top

Ingredients:

    2 oz. organic apricot kernel oil
    7 drops Pink Grapefruit *(Citrus paradisi)*
    5 drops Lemon *(Citrus limon)*
    3 drops May Chang *(Litsea cubeba)*
    5 drops Geranium *(Pelargonium roseum x asperum)*
    5 drops Cypress *(Cupressus sempervirens)*
    3 drops Rosemary *(Rosmarinus officinalis ct. verbenone)*
    2 drops Juniper Berry *(Juniperis communis)*

Directions:

Blend oils in 2 oz. organic apricot kernel oil in glass bottle. Gently rock back and forth to gently mix essential oils with carrier oil and place treatment pump top on. Use 3-4 pumps for the blend for overall massage on arms, legs, torso and neck using upward strokes towards the heart space.

Appendix

Essential Oils at a Glance

This section will give you a more in-depth look at the healing properties essential oils possess for hormone balance. You can use it cross reference with the essential oil remedy mapper in the quick reference guides to hone in on your symptoms and pinpoint the exact oil your body needs. Use it as a guide to learn more about the oils and create your own essential oil blends. This is by no means a complete list of all the essential oils that can make a difference in balancing hormones but it includes the ones that I work with on a daily basis in my practice. Although the oils here have many properties, I have only described their qualities in relationship to hormone balance.

"I am continually impressed with Angela's knowledge of essential oils. She knows how they should be used, what properties each oil has to offer, and how essential oils can enhance everyday living!"

~ Patti

Atlas Cedarwood (*Cedrus atlantica*) - Anti-inflammatory, improves mature skin, improves cellulite, supports healthy hair, nervous system sedative, grounding, supports mood and self esteem, relieves vaginal itching and bladder irritation, water retention, aids varicose veins, supports weight management.

Bergamot (*Citrus bergamia*) - Potent antidepressant, lowers irritability, helps control cholesterol levels, helps control appetite, regulates metabolism and prevents cholesterol absorption, eases PMS, relieves menstrual cramps, leaky bladder, relieves fear & anxiety, improves emotional stability, affects HPA Axis to reduce corticosterone response to stress, balances pineal & pituitary glands for hormone regulation, helps regulate sleep cycles.

Black Spruce (*Picea mariana*) - Adaptogenic to support endocrine system, reduces mental fatigue and burnout, depression, low stamina, supports weight loss, adrenal tonic, pain reliever, aids in menstrual disorders, improves skin, immune enhancer, stimulates thymus gland and regulates pituitary gland, regulates estrogen and progesterone.

Blue Tansy (*Tanacetum annuum*) - Anti-inflammatory, soothes irritability and al stress related conditions, agitated depression, oversensitivity, aids insomnia, acts as a sedative, PMS and pain reliever, aids IBS symptoms, helps balance blood sugar.

Cinnamon bark/leaf (*Cinnamomum zeylanicum*) - Anti-inflammatory, destroys viruses, helps stabilize blood sugar, digestive aid, supports immune health, edema, helps with IBS, anxiety, PMS and insomnia.

Clary Sage (*Salvia sclarea*) - Aphrodisiac, antidepressant, uterine restorative, regulates menstrual periods, eases tension and muscle cramps, helps control cellulite, manages cortisol levels, supports action of estrogen, relieves PMS, eases heart palpitations and hot flashes, may inhibit growth of breast and uterine cancers, soothes anxiety and fatigue, improves sex drive, aids sleep, antidepressant, calms the liver.

Clove (*Eugenia caryophyllata*) - Antidepressant stimulant and aphrodisiac, helps regulate the immune system, pain relief, thyroid balancing, helps prevent blood clots, relieves nervous exhaustion, fatigue and brain fog.

Cypress (*Cupressus sempervirens*) - Strong antioxidant compounds, calms the nervous system, detoxifying, pain reliever, gets rid of excess fluid, relieves bloating, manages perspiration, helps reduce cholesterol levels, relieves hot flashes, tones and strengthens circulatory system, relieves lymphatic congestion, aids in regulating menstrual cycles.

Eucalyptus (*Eucalyptus radiata*) - Anti-inflammatory, supports genitourinary system, can help relieve menstrual cramps, supports blood and lymph flow, strengthens immune function.

Fennel (*Foeniculum vulgare var. dulce*) - Supports liver, kidneys, bladder and digestion, relieves edema, enhances detoxification, relieves cramps and spasms, moves stagnant lymph.

Frankincense (*Boswelli carterii*) - anti-inflammatory, antidepressant, thyroid balancing, lowers cortisol levels, relieves headaches, helps regulate heart rate, grounding, eases anxiety, pain reliever, increases white blood count and supports immune system, balances menstrual cycles and PMS symptoms, anti-aging properties to nourish and renew skin.

Geranium (*Pelargonium roseum x asperum*) - sedative properties, nerve tonic, relieves hot flashes, pain reliever, emotionally uplifting, reduces yeast and fungal infections, eases anxiety and stress, improves mood swings, supports healthy skin, eases heart palpitations, helps with salt cravings and fluid retention, offers blood sugar balance, liver and pelvic decongestant.

German Chamomile (*Matricaria recitita*) - Anti-anxiety, supports emotional stability, improves sleep issues, soothes nerve pain and restless legs, uterine relaxant, digestive aid for IBS, eases PMS as an antispasmodic.

Ginger (*Zingiber officinale*) - Anti-inflammatory, antidepressant, antioxidant, detoxifying, digestive aid, breaks down sugar and help it absorb, circulates blood, warming - helps with cold hands and feet, relieves muscle aches, regulates menstrual cycle, pain reliever, digestive aid, immune regulator.

Green Myrtle (*Myrtus communis*) - Nervous system regulator, digestive aid, menstrual regulator, eases heavy periods, soothes hot flashes, assists hypoglycemia, claustrophobia associated with estrogen levels, eases hypertension.

Holy Basil (*Ocimum sanctum*) - Anti-inflammatory, antidepressant, antiviral (herpes), adaptogen that manages cellular stress, adrenal restorative, eases muscle tension, contains cholesterol-lowering properties, relieves pain, digestive aid, supports thyroid and adrenals.

Jasmine (*Jasminum grandiflorum*) - Uplifts mood, aphrodisiac, calms the mind, relieves depression, uterine restorative, supports healthy skin, eases menstrual pain and cramps, improves sex drive.

Lavender (*Lavandula angustifolia*) - Sedative qualities, relieves tension and stress, shown to reduce cholesterol, relieves menstrual cramps, pain relieving, eases PMS, improves feeling of well being, supports mental alertness, suppresses situational anxiety, reduces headaches, soothes muscle aches, relieves hot flashes, aids leaky bladder, sleep restorative.

Lemon (*Citrus limon*) - Uplifts mood, detoxifying, aids leaky bladder, increases metabolism and burns fat, manages stress and fights depression, reduces and prevents cravings for sweets, increases focus, decreases mental fatigue and brain fog, reduces bloating, liver restorative, supports lymph.

Lemongrass (*Cymbopogon citratus*) - Anti-inflammatory, antidepressant, detoxifying, removes stagnation for lymphatic system, promotes blood circulation and lowers cholesterol levels, reduces mental fatigue, relieves headaches, improves digestion and metabolism, eases IBS, pain reliever.

Linden Blossom (*Tilia vulgaris*) - Reduces anxiety and stress, euphoric, acts as sleep aid, helps regulate blood pressure, detoxifying, liver tonic, digestive aid, reduces headaches, contains antioxidants, diuretic to aid edema, skin restorative.

Mandarin - There are 2 varieties of mandarin, red and green. Red Mandarin or tangerine (*Citrus reticulata*) and Green Mandarin (*Citrus reticulata var. mandarine*). - Soothes and balances blood, circulatory system and heart, calms nervous agitation, promotes sleep, helps manage weight, digestive aid, antispasmodic, moves lymph, supports liver function, calms emotional stress, relieves anxiety and depression.

May Chang (*Litsea cubeba*) - Antidepressant, relaxant, improves mental fatigue and brain fog, uplifting, enhances skin tone, improves digestion, helps manage stress, cools hot flashes, moves lymphatic congestion, reduces heart palpitations.

Melissa (*Melissa officinalis*) - also referred to as Lemon Balm - Anti-inflammatory, relieves anxiety and nervous tension, calming and uplifting, antiviral (herpes), digestive aid, improves brain fog, supports heart function, soothes grief and emotional sensitivity.

Myrrh (*Commiphora myrrha*) - Anti-inflammatory, antioxidant, helps to reduce cholesterol and lower blood pressure, thyroid balancing, endocrine regulator, relieves nervous exhaustion, promotes circulation of blood and lymph, enhances healthy skin, improves immune and digestive systems.

Neroli (*Citrus aurantium*) - Anti-inflammatory, antidepressant, antispasmodic, uplifting yet calming, manages stress, euphoric, aphrodisiac, regulates menstruation, mild sedative, digestive restorative, soothes cramps and eases PMS, helps lower blood pressure, improves skin elasticity.

Nutmeg (*Myristica fragrans*) - Digestive aid, aphrodisiac, reduces mood swings and depression, helps with genitourinary infections, liver detoxifier, supports cardiovascular system, adrenal tonic, assists with sleep issues, relieves menstrual cramps and PMS, pain reliever, promotes hormone balance.

Oregano (*Origanum vulgare*) - Anti-inflammatory, supports immune health, has been shown to reduce cholesterol and triglyceride levels in the blood, powerful antioxidant, used to treat yeast infections, improves gut flora, pain reliever, may have cancer fighting properties, helps with weight loss. <u>Caution:</u> may interact with medications such as blood thinners.

Palmarosa *(Cymbopogon martinii)* - Fights candida overgrowth, balances autonomic system, stimulates hormone production and normalizes thyroid function, treats genito-urinary and reproductive issues such as cystitis, vaginitis, cervicitis and is a uterine tonic, regenerates skin, aids nervous exhaustion and stress related symptoms and promotes feminine strength, stamina & stability, balances cortisol and adrenal function, liver tonic.

Patchouli *(Pogostemon cablin)* - Anti-inflammatory, antidepressant, antiviral, eases edema, soothes adrenal exhaustion, relieves sleep issues, prevents saggy skin, improves sex drive, aphrodisiac, boosts energy, strengthens immune system, detoxifying, stimulates blood flow, kidney tonic, helps eliminate candida.

Peppermint *(Mentha X piperita)* - Adaptogen, anti-inflammatory, relieves menstrual pain, improves brain function, relieves muscle spasms, encourages hair growth, relieves PMS, blood cleanser, moves stagnation, reduce hot flashes, nerve tonic, digestive soother for IBS.

Pine Needle *(Pinus sylvestris)* - Anti-inflammatory, antidepressant, supports adrenals, relieves PMS, reduces pain, supports thyroid and urinary concerns, reduces anxiety, aids in edema, digestive tonic, relieves gall bladder issues, soothes muscle aches.

Pink Grapefruit *(Citrus paradisi)* - Antioxidant, stimulates liver and gall bladder function, reduces sweet cravings, balances leptin, uplifts mood, reduces anxiety and worry, aids PMS, improves sleep, helps digestion, encourages lymph movement.

Roman Chamomile *(Chamaemelum nobilis)* - acts as a sedative, relieves muscle spasms, soothes headache, aids insomnia, eases menstrual cramps and tension, combats anxiety and stress, eases an overactive mind, relieves PMS, manages breast tenderness, supports white blood cell production and strengthens immune system, liver decongestant,

Rose Otto *(Rosa damascena)* - Anti-inflammatory, aphrodisiac, antidepressant, adaptogen and nerve tonic, helps with major life transitions such as menopause, balances emotions, uterine tonic, improves serotonin levels, balances estrogen, harmonizing effect on the heart, restores skin, pain reliever, helps balance blood sugar, eases mood swings, relieves menstrual cramps.

Rosemary (*Rosmarinus officinalis ct. verbenone*) - skin tonic, soothes menstrual cramps, encouraging hair growth, relieves PMS, edema, reduces cellulite, encourages hormone production, regulates menstrual cycles, fortifies liver, gall bladder and heart, manages stress, clears brain fog, helps regenerate cells, may help reduce high blood sugar.

Sandalwood (*Santalum album*) - Antidepressant, aphrodisiac, improves sex drive, euphoric, balances testosterone, grounding, harmonizes emotions, relieves anxiety, sedative and nervine, immune stimulating, skin regenerative properties, helps lower blood pressure.

Sweet Marjoram (*Origanum marjorana*) - Aphrodisiac, adaptogenic, relieves menstrual cramps, gentle sedative, nervous system tonic, quells anger, conflict, agitation and anxiety, mild diuretic, support the heart and circulatory system, eases heart palpitations, relieves urinary pain.

Sweet Orange (*Citrus sinensis*) - Antidepressant, uplifts mood, aids in digestion, improves sleep, relieves nervous anxiety, lowers cortisol, improves skin tone, reduces cellulite, detoxifying for liver and lymph.

Tea Tree (*Melaleuca alternifolia*) - Antibacterial (herpes), eases symptoms of vaginitis, cystitis and candida, supports immune function, fights bladder infections, pain reliever, supports healthy skin, emotionally uplifting.

Thyme (*Thymus vulgaris*) - anti-inflammatory, balances progesterone, thyroid balancing, stimulates the thymus gland, immune protector and supporter with antioxidants, relieves muscles spasms and cramps, relieves fatigue, strengthens nerves, alleviates nervous exhaustion, detoxifying.

Vetiver (*Vetiveria zizanoides*) - Anti-inflammatory, promotes Relief of anxiety, chronic stress and panic, nerve tonic for emotional sensitivity, grounding, sedative relaxant, aids with sleep issues, immune and circulatory stimulant, relieves nervous tension, skin and hair restorative.

Ylang Ylang (*Cananga odorata*) - antidepressant, aphrodisiac, euphoric, reduces blood pressure, relieves anxiety, skin rejuvenating, increases self esteem, relieves PMS, stimulating to liver and endocrine system, supports kidney and adrenal function, regulates an overstimulated nervous system.

Resources List

Where to Find Trusted Quality Essential Oils & Other Ingredients

The best results require the best ingredients. As the Oregon director for the National Association of Holistic Aromatherapists, I have many colleagues who source high quality pure essential oils. There are also sources listed here for carrier oils and bases to make products with.

Trusted Essential Oil Companies

Aromatics International - www.aromatics.com

Cathy Skipper - www.cathysattars.com

Mountain Rose Herbs - www.mountainroseherbs.com

Nature's Sunshine - http://MenopauseSuccess.mynsp.com

Snow Lotus - www.snowlotus.org

Stillpoint Aromatics - www.stillpointaromatics.com

Tiffany Carole - www.bluedolphineo.com and www.monara.org (coming in spring 2019)

Suppliers for Other Ingredients

Amazon - www.amazon.com
Wild yam cream (indian meadow herbals), organic hexane free castor oil (heritage store), wool flannel (heritage store), magnesium flakes (ancient minerals brand), epsom salts.

E.D. Luce packaging - www.essentialsupplies.com
Roll-on bottles, 5ml bottles, 2 oz. bottles, dropper bottles and lids, glass jars, treatment pump lids, sprayer top lids.

Elements Bath and Body - www.elementsbathandbody.com
Roll-on bottles, natural beeswax pastilles, vitamin E, packaging.

Essential Wholesale & Labs - www.essentialwholesale.com
unscented lotion base, carrier oils.

iherb - www.iherb.com - Jarro-Dophilus for women probiotic capsules

Mountain Rose Herbs - www.mountainroseherbs.com
Beeswax pastilles, arnica infused oil, hydrosols, witch hazel, tamanu oil, baobab oil, sweet almond oil, apricot kernel oil, bentonite clay, castile soap, "00" gel capsules, dead sea salt, aloe vera gel, shea butter, fenugreek seeds.

Nature's Sunshine - http://MenopauseSuccess.mynsp.com
Lobelia essence, sunshine concentrate (shower get base), distress remedy homeopathic, MSM cream, silver shield, black ointment, golden salve, vitamin E capsules.

Stillpoint Aromatics - www.stillpointaromatics.com
Blank inhalers, 5ml bottles.

Bibliography

Studies, Research Articles and Websites

Aromatherapy Massage Affects Menopausal Symptoms in Korean Climacteric Women: A Pilot-Controlled Clinical Trial. Using lavender, rose geranium, rose and jasmine essential oils in almond and evening primrose oils for a variety of menopausal symptoms Hur et al.
https://www.ncbi.nlm.nih.gov/pmc/articles/PMC2529395/
accessed 8/20/18

Balance out Your Hormones Naturally
Research data on thyme essential oil and progesterone
Axe, Dr.
Oils with Sharelle, 2015
http://www.oilswithsharelle.com.au/uploads/9/7/3/6/97361762/balance_out_your_hormones_naturally.pdf
accessed 7/6/18

Changes in 5-hydroxytryptamine and cortisol plasma levels in menopausal women after inhalation of clary sage oil. Clary sage essential oil reduces cortisol by 36%
Lee et al.
https://www.ncbi.nlm.nih.gov/pubmed/24802524
accessed 9/26/201

Cholesterol: Friend Or Foe?
Natasha Campbell-McBride MAY 4, 2008
https://www.westonaprice.org/health-topics/know-your-fats/cholesterol-friend-or-foe/
accessed 9/27/18

Common herbs, essential oils, and monoterpenes potently modulate bone metabolism
Pine oil to preserve bone strength in menopause
https://www.thebonejournal.com/article/S8756-3282(03)00027-9/fulltext
accessed 7/6/18

Effects of Aroma Massage on Home Blood Pressure, Ambulatory Blood Pressure, and Sleep Quality in Middle-Aged Women with Hypertension using bergamot, lavender, clary sage essential oils
Myeong Sook Ju et al.
https://www.hindawi.com/journals/ecam/2013/403251/
accessed 8/20/18

Effect of aromatherapy massage on dysmenorrhea in Turkish students.
Apay SE, Arslan S, Akpinar RB, Celebioglu A.
https://www.ncbi.nlm.nih.gov/pubmed/23158705
accessed 10/7/18

Effects of essential oil exposure on salivary estrogen concentration in perimenopausal women.
Shinohara et al.
https://www.ncbi.nlm.nih.gov/pubmed/28326753
accessed 9/14/18

Effect of Inhalation of Aroma of Geranium Essence on Anxiety and Physiological Parameters during First Stage of Labor in Nulliparous Women: a Randomized Clinical Trial.
Rashidi et al.
https://www.ncbi.nlm.nih.gov/pubmed/26161367
accessed 8/14/18

Effects of Inhalation of Essential Oil of Neroli (Citrus aurantium L. var. amara) on Menopausal Symptoms, Stress, and Estrogen in Postmenopausal Women: A Randomized Controlled Trial
Seo Yeon Choi, Purum Kang, Hui Su Lee, Geun Hee Seol et al.
https://www.hindawi.com/journals/ecam/2014/796518/
accessed 7/20/18

Effects of geranium aroma on anxiety among patients with acute myocardial infarction: A triple-blind randomized clinical trial.
Shirzadegan et al.
https://www.ncbi.nlm.nih.gov/pubmed/29122262
accessed 7/6/18

Effect of Aromatherapy on Symptoms of Dysmenorrhea in College Students: A Randomized Placebo-Controlled Clinical Trial
Sun-Hee Han, Myung Haeng Hur, Jane Buckle, Jeeyae Choi, Myeong Soo Lee
Published Online: 2 Aug 2006 https://doi.org/10.1089/acm.2006.12.535
https://www.liebertpub.com/doi/abs/10.1089/acm.2006.12.535
accessed 7/16/18

Effect of orange peel essential oil on postpartum sleep quality: A randomized controlled clinical trial
Mirghafourvand M. Charandabi SMA, Hakimi S, Khoadaie L, Galeshi M. European Journal of Integrative Medicine. 2016;8:62–66.

Essential plant oils and headache mechanisms.
Göbel et al.
Peppermint essential oil for headaches
https://www.ncbi.nlm.nih.gov/pubmed/23196150
accessed 8/20/18

Essential oils used in aromatherapy: A systemic review.
Ali B, Al-Wabel NA, Shams S, Ahamad A, Khan SA, Anwar F.
Asian Pacific Journal of Tropical Biomedicine. 2015;5(8):601–611.
https://www.sciencedirect.com/science/article/pii/S2221169115001033
accessed 10/7/18

Estrogen and progestin bioactivity of foods, herbs, and spices.
Zava et al.
Progesterone balancing effects of Thyme essential oil
https://www.ncbi.nlm.nih.gov/pubmed/9492350
accessed 8/20/18

Facts about the Thyroid Gland and Thyroid Disease
The American Thyroid Association (ATA)
https://www.thyroid.org/media-main/press-room/
accessed 9/26/18

Hypoglycemic and antioxidant effects of leaf essential oil of Pelargonium graveolens L'Hér. in alloxan induced diabetic rats.
Boukhris et al.
https://www.ncbi.nlm.nih.gov/pubmed/22734822
accessed 9/6/18

Impact of lemongrass oil, an essential oil, on serum cholesterol.
Elson et al.
https://www.ncbi.nlm.nih.gov/pubmed/2586227
accessed 9/27/18

In vitro anti-diabetic effect and chemical component analysis of 29 essential oils products.
Yen et al.
https://www.ncbi.nlm.nih.gov/pubmed/28911435
accessed 7/22/18

Menopause: Understanding and managing the transition using essential oils vs. traditional allopathic medicine
Melissa A. Clanton
https://achs.edu/mediabank/files/melissa_clanton.pdf
accessed 9/26/18

Oregano essential oil properties in relationship to estrogen and breast cancer
Arunasree
https://www.ncbi.nlm.nih.gov/pubmed/20096548
https://www.healthline.com/nutrition/9-oregano-oil-benefits-and-uses#section11
https://www.ncbi.nlm.nih.gov/pubmed/20096548
accessed 10/7/18

Oxytocin: The Hormone of Love
Dr. Tarman Aziz
http://creativehealthinstituteusa.com/2017/02/28/oxytocin-hormone-love/   accessed 9/26/18

Peppermint promotes hair growth without toxic signs
Ji Young Oh et al.
https://www.ncbi.nlm.nih.gov/pmc/articles/PMC4289931/
accessed 9/26/18

Presentation and Management of Major Depressive Disorder in Perimenopausal and Postmenopausal Women
Clayton & Ninan
https://www.ncbi.nlm.nih.gov/pmc/articles/PMC2882813/
accessed 7/6/18

Progesterone and Menopausal Symptoms
Women in Balance Institute
National University of Natural Medicine
https://womeninbalance.org/2014/09/19/the-anatomy-of-a-hot-flash/
accessed 9/26/18

Role of Estrogen in Thyroid Function and Growth Regulation
Santin & Furlanetto
https://www.ncbi.nlm.nih.gov/pmc/articles/PMC3113168/
accessed 9/25/18

Self-aromatherapy massage of the abdomen for the reduction of menstrual pain and anxiety during menstruation in nurses: A placebo-controlled clinical trial.
Marzouk et al.
https://www.ncbi.nlm.nih.gov/pmc/articles/PMC3638625/
accessed 9/13/18

Study in Tunisia demonstrated geranium's ability to decrease blood glucose levels
Boukhris et al.
https://www.ncbi.nlm.nih.gov/pmc/articles/PMC3439344/
accessed 9/6/18

Study using palmarosa and geranium essential oils for effective stress reduction
Andrade et al.
https://www.ncbi.nlm.nih.gov/pmc/articles/PMC4276358/
accessed 8/6/18

The Benefits of Thymus Vulgaris
By Cathy Wong, ND | Reviewed by Richard N. Fogoros, MD
Updated September 21, 2018
https://www.verywellhealth.com/the-benefits-of-thymus-vulgaris-88803
accessed 8/20/18

The Effect of Lavender Aromatherapy on Autonomic Nervous System in Midlife Women with Insomnia
Li-Wei Chien et al.
https://www.hindawi.com/journals/ecam/2012/740813/
accessed 7/6/18

The Effectiveness of Aromatherapy in Reducing Pain: A Systematic Review and Meta-Analysis
Shaheen E. Lakhan et al.
https://www.ncbi.nlm.nih.gov/pmc/articles/PMC5192342/
accessed 8/14/18

The Relationship Between Adrenal Function and Menopausal Symptoms
menopause statistics
https://ndnr.com/womens-health/the-relationship-between-adrenal-function-and-menopausal-symptoms-2/
accessed 9/29/18

Top 10 essential oils for hormone balance
https://www.gurunanda.com/blogs/aromatherapy/top-10-essential-oils-for-hormone-balance
accessed 9/26/18

Therapeutic qualities of linden blossom essential oil
http://www.yogawiz.com/aromatherapy/aromatherapy-essential-oils/linden-blossom-essential-oil.html
accessed 10/7/18

Top 3 Essential Oils to Balance Hormones Naturally
Dr. Axe
https://draxe.com/essential-oils-for-hormones/
accessed 6/19/17

What You Should Know About Your Thyroid and Menopause
Neel Duggal. Medically reviewed by Debra Rose Wilson, PhD, MSN, RN, IBCLC, AHN-BC, CHT on May 19, 2017
https://www.healthline.com/health/menopause/thyroid-and-menopause#estrogen
accessed 9/26/18

Books, Presentations, Classes

Balas, Kimberly, ND, *Applied Aromatherapy*
2002

Battaglia, Salvatore, *The Complete Guide to Aromatherapy*
Perfect Potion, 1995

Berkowsky, Dr. Bruce - Joseph Ben Hi-Meyer Research, Inc. 2012-2013 SPE Repertory of Essential Oils pages 21, 96, 100, 103

Bieler, Henry G. Food Is Your Best Medicine: *The Pioneering Nutrition Classic*
Ballantine Books, 1982

Carole, Tiffany - Master Healers retreat presentations
The soul opening energetics of essential oils with specific acu-points
Duvall, WA 2018 www.tiffanycarole.com

Fifield, Bill. *Integrated Guide to Essential Oils & Aromatherapy*
Sound Concepts, 2nd edition 2014.

Gittleman, Ann Louise, PhD, *Before the Change: Taking charge of your perimenopause*
HarperCollins, revised and updated 2017

Hochell, Jennifer, *JennScents Aromatherapy Custom Blending Bar Business Guide*
Jennscents, Inc., 2005

Holmes, Peter, Aromatica: *A clinical guide to essential oil therapeutics, volume 1: Principles and Profiles*
Singing Dragon, 2016

Holmes, Peter, *Clinical Aromatherapy: Using essential oils for healing body & soul*
Tiger Lily Press, 2001

Horne, Steven and Easley, Thomas, *Modern Herbal Medicine*
The school of modern herbal medicine, 2014

Jones, Larissa, *Aromatherapy for Body, Mind & Spirit*
Evergreen Aromatherapy, 2002

Klements, Cindy - Hormones and Women's Health
Nature's Sunshine Products convention presentation 2011

Northrup, Christiane M.D. - *Women's Bodies, Women's Wisdom*
Bantam Books, 2010

Northrup, Christiane M.D. - *Goddesses Never Age*
Hay House, Inc., 2015

Northrup, Christiane M.D. - *The Wisdom of Menopause*
Bantam Books, revised edition 2006

Pressimone, Jennifer, *Jennscents Holistic Aromatherapy Comprehensive Guide*
Jennscents, Inc., 2015

Price, Shirley and Len, *Aromatherapy for Health Professionals*
Elsevier Ltd., 3rd edition 1995

Rose, Jeanne, *The Aromatherapy Book – Applications and Inhalations*
North Atlantic Books,1992

Schnaubelt, Kurt, *The Healing Intelligence of Essential Oils: The Science of Advanced Aromatherapy*
Healing Arts Press, 1998

Snyder, Dr. Mariza, *Smart Mom's Guide to Essential Oils: Natural Solutions for a healthy family, toxin-free home and happier you*
Ulysses Press, 2017

Stiles, K.G., *The essential oils complete reference guide: over 250 recipes for natural wholesome aromatherapy*
Page Street Publishing, 2017

The Menopause Guidebook
The North American Menopause Society (NAMS)
8th edition 2015

Tisserand, Robert, *The Art of Aromatherapy*
C. W. Daniel, 1977

Ward, Mary & Birk-Schneider, Victoria-Marie, *Aromatherapy, The Scent of Life*
V.M. & M., 2010

Wszelaki, Magdalena, *Cooking for Hormone Balance*
HarperCollins, 2018

About The Author

Angela Sidlo is passionate about health and wellness. For the past 12 years her focus has been helping women worldwide, find balance in body mind and spirit using essential oils. She holds certifications in holistic aromatherapy, health coaching, reflexology and reiki, bringing this unique foundational skill set into her practice. As a Menopause Success coach, Through her own experience of going through menopause, Angela uniquely holds space for women to make beautiful transformational shifts to reclaim their vibrancy in the wisdom years with ease and grace. She gently guides women to make small changes and become co-creators for big results in finding hormonal balance.

In her practice she offers public speaking, one-on-one coaching programs, small group workshops, retreats and supportive online programs. These include the 14 Day Hormone Balance Detox, Aromatherapy: The Gateway to Happy Hormones course and the Menopause Success mastery program.

She currently serves as the Oregon Director for the National Association of Holistic Aromatherapists, teaches aromatherapy at the Oregon School of Massage, formulates essential oil blends for Columbia Memorial Hospital in Astoria, Oregon and has her own line of Menopause Success health and beauty products. Angela is also co-author of *The Silver Linings Storybook* and author of *Endless Pastabilities Cookbook*.

Connect with Angela

www.AngelaSidlo.com

https://www.facebook.com/angela.sidlo

https://www.facebook.com/groups/846107975572992/

https://www.instagram.com/menopausesuccesscoach/

Index

GHRH, 23
Ginger, 57, 121, 123, 153
glucagon, 23
glucocorticoids, 23
Green Mandarin, 59, 64, 65, 131, 154–155
Green Myrtle, 57, 121, 154

H

hair and skincare essentials, 110–120
Hashimoto's disease, 40
HDL cholesterol, effect of increased insulin levels
    on, 37, 44
headache relief, 94
heart, as part of endocrine system, 21
Helichrysum, 91, 115, 116, 122
hippocampus, as part of olfactory pathway, 19
histamine, 23
Holy Basil, 34, 57, 64, 68, 69, 94, 129, 146, 154
hormone balance, multifaceted approach as
    needed to find, 16
hormone replacement therapy
    cautions with, 28
    as not offering sustainable solutions, 9
hormones. *See also specific hormones*
    illustration of where they are produced in body, 23
    ones that are major players regarding
        peri-menopause and menopause, 22
    ones that are minor players regarding
        peri-menopause and menopause, 23
    produced by endocrine system, 21–22
    role of, 17
    satiation hormone, 53
    steroid hormones, 43
hot flashes
    anatomy of, 47
    explained, 46–48
    percent of women as experiencing, 61
    taking control of, 81–86
hydrosol, defined, 18
hyperinsulinemia, 36
hypothalamus
    as master regulator for hormones, 40
    as part of endocrine system, 22

as part of olfactory pathway, 18, 19
    production of hormones by, 23
hypothyroidism, 37, 38, 39
Hyssop, 99

I

IGF, 23
immune enhancement, 148–150
inflammation, hyperinsulinemia as major con-
    tributor of, 36
inhalation, as application method, 19, 20
inhalers
    Anxiety Free Aroma Inhaler, 62
    Appetite Control Aroma Inhaler, 107
    Craving Calmer Aroma Inhaler, 105
    Depression Free Aroma Inhaler, 61
    De-Stress This Mess Aroma Inhaler, 75
    Emotional Calm Aroma Inhaler, 65
    Emotional Calming Aroma Inhaler, 72
    Energize Me Aroma Inhaler, 76
    Fatigue Fighter Aroma Inhaler, 77
    Immune Support Aroma Inhaler, 148
    Radical Focus Aroma Inhaler, 68
    Sleep Ease Aroma Inhaler, 95
    Weight Away Aroma Inhaler, 109
inhibin, 23
insulin
    basics of, 36–38
    hormone that is major player regarding
        peri-menopause and menopause, 22
    production of, 23
    signs of high insulin (insulin resistance), 38
insulin resistance, 37, 38, 44
intestines, as part of endocrine system, 21
intimacy, improvement of, 101–103

J

Jasmine, 45, 57, 66, 101, 102, 137, 154
Juniper Berry, 136, 150

K

Kaffir Lime, 63, 66